*Medical Terminology*

# Word Builder and Communications

# WORKBOOK

# Other Related Titles from McGraw-Hill

McGraw-Hill's Medical Dictionary for Allied Health 1e, 007-334727-2

Medical Language for Modern Health Care 1e, 007-327294-9

Medical Terminology: A Programmed Approach 1e, 007-333505-3

Medical Terminology: Language for Health Care 2e, 007-327295-7

Medical Terminology Essentials 1e, 007-325644-7

Introduction to Medical Terminology 1e, 007-302261-6

*Medical Terminology*

# Word Builder and Communications

# WORKBOOK

## Nina Thierer, CMA, BS, CPC, CCAT
*Ivy Tech Community College of Indiana*
*Fort Wayne, IN*

## Kevin Dumith

 **Higher Education**

Boston   Burr Ridge, IL   Dubuque, IA   New York   San Francisco   St. Louis
Bangkok   Bogotá   Caracas   Kuala Lumpur   Lisbon   London   Madrid   Mexico City
Milan   Montreal   New Delhi   Santiago   Seoul   Singapore   Sydney   Taipei   Toronto

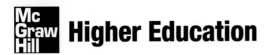

# Higher Education

MEDICAL TERMINOLOGY WORD BUILDER AND COMMUNICATIONS WORKBOOK

Published by McGraw-Hill, a business unit of The McGraw-Hill Companies, Inc., 1221 Avenue of the Americas, New York, NY 10020. Copyright " 2008 by The McGraw-Hill Companies, Inc. All rights reserved. No part of this publication may be reproduced or distributed in any form or by any means, or stored in a database or retrieval system, without the prior written consent of The McGraw-Hill Companies, Inc., including, but not limited to, in any network or other electronic storage or transmission, or broadcast for distance learning.McGraw-Hill Companies, Inc., including, but not limited to, in any network or other electronic storage or transmission, or broadcast for distance learning.

Some ancillaries, including electronic and print components, may not be available to customers outside the United States.

This book is printed on recycled, acid-free paper containing 10% postconsumer waste.

1 2 3 4 5 6 7 8 9 0 QPD/QPD 0 9 8 7

ISBN 978–0–07–340192–8
MHID 0–07–340192–7

Publisher: *David T. Culverwell*
Senior Sponsoring Editor: *Thomas E. Casson*
Developmental Editor: *Lorraine K. Buczek*
Senior Marketing Manager: *Nancy Bradshaw*
Senior Project Manager: *Kay J. Brimeyer*
Senior Production Supervisor: *Sherry L. Kane*
Designer: *Laurie B. Janssen*
Cover Design: *Studio Montage*
Compositor: *Techbooks*
Typeface: *10/12 Melior*
Printer: *Quebecor World Dubuque, IA*

www.mhhe.com

# Contents

# Introduction

The *McGraw-Hill Word Building and Communication Workbook* is designed to test and enhance your skills in understanding medical terminology and its use in communication in health care. The units are arranged so that you build on your knowledge as you use this workbook. This workbook has ample space for you to write in your answers. There is also a companion website that contains allied health documents, career tips, and much more.

The first unit covers the basics of word building as well as some general topics in allied health. In this unit, you are introduced to some sample documents. The medical documents and letters are ones that are commonly found in the health care workplace. The career documents are geared to helping you practice communication skills needed to get a job.

The second unit covers prefixes that will be combined with the word parts in later chapters to form medical terms. Unit 3 covers suffixes that will be used in the same way. As you learn word parts, it is important that you concentrate on including each word part as a permanent part of your vocabulary. Any word parts that you struggle with should be made into flashcards (see the section in this front matter, "Making Flashcards"). The group of flashcards you have at the end of each unit will give you a terrific study tool.

The word parts are the key to understanding many more medical terms than you will have learned individually. This is because most medical terms are built-up words. The following examples of word parts and how they are used should help you understand the basic word-building process.

- A **word root** is the portion of the word that contains its basic meaning. For example, the word root *cardi* means "heart."

  Some other examples of common medical word roots are:
  *dent,* tooth
  *gastr,* stomach
  *laryng,* larynx
  *rhin,* nose
  *ven,* vein

- **Combining forms** are the word root that can be connected to another word part. In some cases, a combining vowel is needed to connect word parts. For example, the word root *cardi* + the combining vowel *o* can form words that relate to the basic meaning "heart," such as *cardiology,* the medical practice involved with studying, diagnosing, and treating disorders of the heart.

  Some other examples of words form from combining forms are:
  *dentalgia*: dent-, tooth + -algia, pain = toothache
  *gastrodynia*: gastr-, stomach + combining vowel −o- + -dynia, pain = stomach ache
  *laryngoplasty*: laryng-, larynx + -o- + -plasty, plastic surgery = plastic surgery on the larynx
  *rhinitis*: rhin-, nose + -it is, inflammation = nose inflammation or runny nose

*venogram*: ven-, vein + -o- + -gram, written record = x-ray image of a vein

- **Prefixes** are word parts attached to the beginning of a word or word root that modify its meaning. For example, the prefix *peri-,* meaning "around, near, surrounding," helps to form the word *pericardium,* meaning "around or surrounding the heart."

  Some other examples of words formed from prefixes are:
  *disinfection:* dis-, apart + infection, infection = removal of infection or sterilization
  *retroperitoneum*: retro-, behind + peritoneum, peritoneum = the space behind the peritoneum

- **Suffixes** are word parts attached to the end of a word or word root that modify its meaning. For example, the suffix *–oid,* meaning "like or resembling," helps to form the word *fibroid,* meaning "made of fibrous tissue."

  Some other examples of words formed from suffixes are:
  *gastrectomy*: gastr-, stomach + -ectomy, removal of = removal of the stomach
  *laryngoscope*: laryng-, larynx + -o- + -scope, tool for examining = device for examining the larynx

Units 4 through 16 are the body system units. Most medical terminology courses are taught by body system and these units are meant to reinforce that learning. Each unit offers practice in word building, proofreading, using an allied health dictionary, and writing, listening, and speaking in the health care setting.

Unit 17 covers pharmacology. The field of pharmacology uses abbreviations extensively. This is the area where most medical errors occur. Make sure to read the introduction to Appendix B, "Medical Errors and Abbreviations," before beginning your review. It is important that you keep the material in the appendix introduction uppermost in your mind whenever you are studying or working in health care. You may find yourself in situations that demand accuracy or they may threaten someone's life or health. Familiarity with pharmacological abbreviations is essential for anyone working in areas that deal with prescriptions and the administration of medication and the giving of medication instructions.

Unit 18 is an overall review of medical terminology. Once you complete the exercises in this workbook successfully, you will have mastered the basics of medical terminology.

There are six appendices in this workbook. Appendix A is a comprehensive list of word parts (combining forms, prefixes, and suffixes). Appendix B, "Medical Errors and Abbreviations," discusses the issue of medical errors and lists many medical abbreviations. Appendix C is an overview of laboratory testing and gives normal test values for many common medical tests. Appendix D is an overview of Complementary and Alternative Medicine (CAM) which may or may not be studied in your medical terminology course. However, many students wind up working in CAM. Also, it is estimated that over 40 percent of the U.S. population uses some form of CAM, so it is a subject you will want to understand. Appendix E is a list of common medical terms with their Spanish translations. Appendix F is a list of Internet Resources.

## Making Flashcards

Medical terminology involves memorization. Flashcards are an effective memorization tool. You can make flashcards using heavy paper or index cards or you can make them online. On the front of a card put a word part that you missed in an exercise or one that you find particularly difficult. On the reverse side of the card, put the meaning and two or three examples of words in which that part appears. You can collect these cards as a group or by separate body systems. Either way, use them repeatedly to test yourself.

## Reviewers

We would like to acknowledge the following individuals for their insightful reviews which contributed to the publication of this workbook:

Diana E. Alagna RN, CPT, RMA
*Branford Hall Career Institute*

Ramona F. Atiles
Allied Health Program Chair
*Career Institute of Health and Technology*

Marsha Cayton, RN, MSN, CPNP, RMA
Medical Assisting Program Manager
*King's College*

Claire E. Maday-Travis, MA, MBA, CPHQ
Director of Allied Health Programs
*The Salter School*

Darlene A. Nelson, M.A.T.
*Gibbs College*

Stephanie J. Suddendorf, CMA, A.A.S
*Thompson Institute*

Sandra E. Walsh, M.S., M.Ed
Director of Education
*ECPI College of Technology*

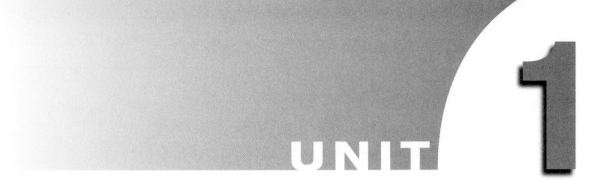

# Communication Using Medical Terms

## How Medical Terms Are Formed

Communication in allied health requires knowledge of many medical terms. Remembering all those terms and their meanings is a very tall order even for the most experienced allied health worker. Fortunately, most medical terms are "built up." This means that they are made up of word parts which have meaning. The four kinds of word parts are the following:

1. **Word roots** are the fundamental part of a word that contains the basic meaning. For example, the word root *cardi-* means "heart."
2. **Combining forms** are the word root and a combining vowel that enable two parts to be connected. For example, the word root *cardi-* plus the combining vowel -o- can form words such as *cardiology,* the medical specialty concerned with the heart.
3. **Prefixes** are word parts that attach to the beginning of a word or word roots to modify the meaning of that word root. For example, *pericardium,* meaning "around the heart" includes the prefix *peri-,* around.
4. **Suffixes** are word parts that attach to the end of a word or word root to modify the meaning of that word root. For example, *fibroid,* meaning "made of fibrous tissue" includes the suffix *-oid,* meaning "like" or "resembling."

Practicing word building will give you the skill to understand many medical terms even if you have never seen them before. The allied health workplace will require you to speak, hear, and write many medical terms. In this workbook, you will practice building medical terms and using them in written medical documents.

## The Systems of the Body

The human body is generally divided into 13 systems. Listed below are the systems and the units in which they are covered in this workbook. For each system, a couple of frequently used combining forms (along with the typical combining vowel shown in parentheses) are given.

1. **Integumentary System**—Unit 4. Includes the skin. Some combining forms are derm(o), dermat(o), skin; pil(o), hair; and onych(o), nail.
2. **Musculoskeletal System**—Unit 5. Includes bones, muscles, and joints. Some combining forms are oste(o), bone; my(o)-, muscle; and arthr(o)-, joint.
3. **Cardiovascular System**—Unit 6. Includes the heart and blood vessels. Some combining forms are cardi(o), heart; angi(o), blood vessel; arteri(o), artery; phleb(o), vein; and vas(o), vein.
4. **Respiratory System**—Unit 7. Includes the respiratory tract and lungs. Some combining forms are pneum(o), pneumon(o), lungs; nas(o), nose; and or(o), mouth.
5. **Nervous System**—Unit 8 includes the brain and spinal cord. Some combining forms are encephal(o), brain; spin(o), spine; and neur(o), nerve.

1

6. **Urinary System**—Unit 9. Includes the kidneys, bladder, and urinary tract. Some combining forms are nephr(o), kidney; ur(o), urine; and cyst(o), bladder.

7. **Female Reproductive System**—Unit 10. Includes the female genitalia and the breasts. Some combining forms are gynec(o), female; uter(o), uterus; and mamm(o), breast.

8. **Male Reproductive System**—Unit 11. Includes the male genitalia. Some combining forms are andr(o), male; orchid(o), testes; and sperm(o), spermat(o), sperm.

9. **Blood System**—Unit 12. Includes the blood circulating throughout the body. Some combining forms are hem(o), blood; erythr(o), red; and leuk(o), white.

10. **Lymphatic and Immune Systems**—Unit 13. Includes the lymph, lymph vessels and organs, and the body's immune systems. Some combining forms are lymph(o), lymph; immun(o), immunity; and tox(o), poison.

11. **Digestive System**—Unit. 14. Includes the digestive tract from the mouth down through the stomach and intestines to the anus, as well as the organs of digestion. Some combining forms are hepat(o), liver; gastr(o), stomach; and enter(o), intestines.

12. **Endocrine System**—Unit 15. Includes the endocrine glands that are the body's master regulators. Some combining forms are adren(o), adrenal glands; pancreat(o), pancreas; and thyroid(o), thyroid.

13. **Sensory System**—Unit 16. Includes the eyes and ears. Some combining forms are ot(o), ear; audi(o), hearing; and opthalm(o), eye.

## Exercises in Word Building

Using the combining forms listed above, as well as the lists of prefixes and suffixes in Units 2 and 3, build 7 words for each body system. You may combine word parts from several body systems. Give the parts of each word and a definition for the built-up word. You may also use the first three sheets of flashcards bound in with this workbook. Make sure to use both prefixes and suffixes and try to build some words with at least three parts. For example:

gastr-, stomach + -algia, pain = gastralgia, stomach pain or stomachache

cardio-, heart + myo-, muscle + -pathy, disease = cardiomyopathy, disease of the heart muscle

### Integumentary System

1. _____

2. _____

3. _____

4. _____

5. _____

6. _____

7. _____

## Musculoskeletal System

1. _____
2. _____
3. _____
4. _____
5. _____
6. _____
7. _____

## Cardiovascular System

1. _____
2. _____
3. _____
4. _____
5. _____
6. _____
7. _____

## Respiratory System

1. _____
2. _____
3. _____
4. _____
5. _____
6. _____
7. _____

## Nervous System

1. _____
2. _____
3. _____
4. _____
5. _____
6. _____
7. _____

## Urinary System

1. _____
2. _____
3. _____
4. _____
5. _____
6. _____
7. _____

## Female Reproductive System

1. _____
2. _____
3. _____
4. _____
5. _____
6. _____
7. _____

## Male Reproductive System

1. _____

2. _____

3. _____

4. _____

5. _____

6. _____

7. _____

## Blood System

1. _____

2. _____

3. _____

4. _____

5. _____

6. _____

7. _____

## Lymphatic and Immune System

1. _____

2. _____

3. _____

4. _____

5. _____

6. _____

7. _____

## Digestive System

1. _____
2. _____
3. _____
4. _____
5. _____
6. _____
7. _____

## Endocrine System

1. _____
2. _____
3. _____
4. _____
5. _____
6. _____
7. _____

## Sensory System

1. _____
2. _____
3. _____
4. _____
5. _____
6. _____
7. _____

## Legal and Ethical Issues

Another aspect of work in allied health is knowing the legal and ethical boundaries that govern medical work. Communications in the medical setting must be guarded carefully both for legal considerations and for the ethical concerns of a patient's right to privacy. The major legal and ethical standards are contained in two things:

1. The American Hospital Association's *Patient's Bill of Rights* lists the basic ways in which patients and their information are to be treated. In communicating medical information you will have to evaluate how your actions fit into the methods you are using both for written and spoken communication.

> The right to considerate and respectful care.
>
> - The right to relevant, current, and understandable information about their diagnosis, treatment, and prognosis.
> - The right to make decisions about the planned care and the right to refuse care.
> - The right to have an advance directive (such as a living will) concerning treatment if they become incapacitated.
> - The right to privacy in all procedures, examinations, and discussions of treatment.
> - The right to confidential handling of all information and records about their care.
> - The right to look over and have all records about their care explained.
> - The right to suggest changes in the planned care or to transfer to another facility.
> - The right to be informed about the business relationships among the hospital and other facilities that are part of the treatment and care.
> - The right to decide whether to take part in experimental treatments.
> - The right to understand their care options after a hospital stay.
> - The right to know about the hospital's policies for settling disputes and to receive and examine an explanation of all charges.

2. HIPAA (the Health Insurance Portability and Accountability Act) was passed in 1966 by Congress. Aside from insurance issues, the law sets standards for the security and privacy of health care data.

The communication practice in this workbook includes some common-sense ways to handle legal and ethical issues that may arise. Refer to the *Patient's Bill of Rights* if you have a question.

## Communication in Health Care

Communication involves speaking, listening, and writing. All three types of communication require courtesy, accuracy, and attention to the rules of privacy. Courtesy is the basic way that all human interaction is made easier and more pleasant. Throughout this workbook, you will work in case study situations that require you to work out realistic interactions with clients and patients. The prime rule to remember is to treat others as you would want to be treated.

Some communications involve creating letters, filling in forms, or working on other documents. The samples shown here can be used in the exercises later in this workbook.

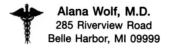

**Alana Wolf, M.D.**
285 Riverview Road
Belle Harbor, MI 09999

March 12, 20XX

Dr. Robert Johnson
16 Tyler Court
Newtown, MI 09990

Dear Dr. Johnson

I saw Laura Spinoza on March the 7th for evaluation of her fibromyalgia. I reviewed her history with her and discussed her treatment for depression. The history suggests that there has not been any new development of an inflammatory rheumatic disease process within the last two years. She does have right thumb-carpal pain, which represents some osteoarthritis. Headaches are frequent but she is receiving no specific therapy. Her sleep pattern remains disturbed at times.

Her height was 62 inches, her weight was 170 lbs, while her BP ws 162/100 in the right arm in the reclining position. Pelvic and rectal examinations were not done. The abdominal examination revealed some mild tenderness in the right lower quadrant without other abnormalities. The musculoskeletal examination revealed rotation and flexion to the left with no other cervical abnormalities. The reminder of the musculo-skeletal examination revealed hypermobility in the elbow and knees and slight bony osteoarthritic enlargement of the thumb-carpal joint. Slight deformity was noted in the right knee with mild patellar-femoral crepitus. Severe bilateral pas planus was present, with the right foot more involved than the left, and ankle vagus deformity with mild bony osteoarthritic enlargement of both 1st MTP joints.

Hope these thoughts are helpful. I want to thank you for the consultation. If I can be of future service with her or other rheumatic-problem patients, please do not hesitate to conta t me.

*Alana Wolf, MD*

Alana ' M.D.

May 21, 2008

Pediatric Associates
745 Main Street
Summers, Illinois 88888

Attn: Office Manager

Dear Sir or Madam:

I was very interested to see your advertisement for a medical assistant in the *Chicago Sun Times* (5-19-08). I have been seeking just such an opportunity as this, and I think my background and your requirements may be a good match. My resume is enclosed for your review.  As you can see, I will have finished my certification examination on July 1 and am seeking full-time employment. I will follow up next week with a call to answer any questions and to schedule an interview at your convenience.

In addition, I was a volunteer at a local hospital during the last three summers. During that time, I learned to deal with patients, respect the privacy of records and of individuals, and had extensive experience answering the phone in a courteous and helpful manner. The experience was extremely rewarding and led to my decision to pursue a career in health care.

Thank you for your attention to these materials. I certainly look forward to exploring this further.

Yours truly,

*Melanie Rodriguez*

Melanie Rodriguez

Enclosure

Melanie Rodriguez
14 South Allenwood Street
Summers, Illinois 88888

(111) 222-3333

| | |
|---|---|
| OBJECTIVE: | Medical Assistant position in the greater Chicago area. |
| SUMMARY: | Will graduate in June from Summers Career College with a degree in medical assisting. Will take certification examination on July 1. Two years of varied part-time job experience. Proficient with MS Office, Windows 2000/XP, and the Internet. |
| EDUCATION: | Summers Career College, certificate in medical assisting, June, 2008. |
| EXPERIENCE: | Summers Convalescent Center, August 2007-present. Part-time receptionist. Duties include greeting patients and visitors, telephone answering, and some office clerk duties.<br>        McDonald's (During high School). Part-time counter job, eventually promoted to assistant store manager. Received Employee of the Month award twice. |
| ACTIVITIES: | • Volunteer, American Red Cross, Summers Animal Rescue Center. |

---

MEDICARE NATIONWIDE
1000 HIGH ST
TOLEDO, OH 43601-0213

| 1500 |
|---|

**HEALTH INSURANCE CLAIM FORM**

APPROVED BY NATIONAL UNIFORM CLAIM COMMITTEE 08/05

☐☐ PICA      PICA ☐☐☐

1. MEDICARE  MEDICAID  TRICARE CHAMPUS  CHAMPVA  GROUP HEALTH PLAN  FECA BLK LUNG  OTHER    1a. INSURED'S I.D. NUMBER      (For Program in Item 1)
☒ (Medicare #)  ☐ (Medicaid #)  ☐ (Sponsor's SSN)  ☐ (Member ID#)  ☐ (SSN or ID)  ☐ (SSN)  ☐ (ID)
**302461884A**

2. PATIENT'S NAME (Last Name, First Name, Middle Initial)    3. PATIENT'S BIRTH DATE   MM DD YY   SEX    4. INSURED'S NAME (Last Name, First Name, Middle Initial)
**HUANG ERIC**    03 13 1940 M☒ F☐

5. PATIENT'S ADDRESS (No., Street)    6. PATIENT RELATIONSHIP TO INSURED    7. INSURED'S ADDRESS (No., Street)
**1109 BAUER ST**    Self ☒ Spouse ☐ Child ☐ Other ☐

CITY **SHAKER HEIGHTS**   STATE **OH**    8. PATIENT STATUS    CITY    STATE
   Single ☐ Married ☒ Other ☐

ZIP CODE **44118 6789**   TELEPHONE (Include Area Code) **(555) 639 1787**    Employed ☐ Full-Time Student ☐ Part-Time Student ☐    ZIP CODE    TELEPHONE (INCLUDE AREA CODE) ( )

9. OTHER INSURED'S NAME (Last Name, First Name, Middle Initial)    10. IS PATIENT'S CONDITION RELATED TO:    11. INSURED'S POLICY GROUP OR FECA NUMBER **NONE**

a. OTHER INSURED'S POLICY OR GROUP NUMBER    a. EMPLOYMENT? (CURRENT OR PREVIOUS) ☐ YES ☒ NO    a. INSURED'S DATE OF BIRTH MM DD YY   SEX M☐ F☐

b. OTHER INSURED'S DATE OF BIRTH MM DD YY   SEX M☐ F☐    b. AUTO ACCIDENT? ☐ YES ☒ NO   PLACE (State)    b. EMPLOYER'S NAME OR SCHOOL NAME

c. EMPLOYER'S NAME OR SCHOOL NAME    c. OTHER ACCIDENT? ☐ YES ☒ NO    c. INSURANCE PLAN NAME OR PROGRAM NAME

d. INSURANCE PLAN NAME OR PROGRAM NAME    10d. RESERVED FOR LOCAL USE    d. IS THERE ANOTHER HEALTH BENEFIT PLAN? ☐ YES ☐ NO   If yes, return to and complete item 9 a-d.

READ BACK OF FORM BEFORE COMPLETING & SIGNING THIS FORM.
12. PATIENT'S OR AUTHORIZED PERSON'S SIGNATURE I authorize the release of any medical or other information necessary to process this claim. I also request payment of government benefits either to myself or to the party who accepts assignment below.

SIGNED **SIGNATURE ON FILE**   DATE _____

13. INSURED'S OR AUTHORIZED PERSON'S SIGNATURE I authorize payment of medical benefits to the undersigned physician or supplier for services described below.

SIGNED _____

14. DATE OF CURRENT: MM DD YY **10 09 2008**   ILLNESS (First symptom) OR INJURY (Accident) OR PREGNANCY(LMP)    15. IF PATIENT HAS HAD SAME OR SIMILAR ILLNESS. GIVE FIRST DATE MM DD YY    16. DATES PATIENT UNABLE TO WORK IN CURRENT OCCUPATION FROM MM DD YY TO MM DD YY

17. NAME OF REFERRING PHYSICIAN OR OTHER SOURCE    17a.   17b. NPI    18. HOSPITALIZATION DATES RELATED TO CURRENT SERVICES FROM MM DD YY TO MM DD YY

19. RESERVED FOR LOCAL USE    20. OUTSIDE LAB? ☐ YES ☒ NO   $ CHARGES

21. DIAGNOSIS OR NATURE OF ILLNESS OR INJURY. (Relate Items 1,2,3 or 4 to Item 24e by Line)
1. **782 . 4** ← Diagnosis code    3. ____ . ____
2. ____ . ____    4. ____ . ____

22. MEDICAID RESUBMISSION CODE   ORIGINAL REF. NO.
23. PRIOR AUTHORIZATION NUMBER

| 24. A. DATE(S) OF SERVICE | | | | | | B. PLACE OF SERVICE | C. EMG | D. PROCEDURES, SERVICES, OR SUPPLIES (Explain Unusual Circumstances) CPT/HCPCS \| MODIFIER | E. DIAGNOSIS POINTER | F. $ CHARGES | G. DAYS OR UNITS | H. EPSDT Family Plan | I. ID. QUAL. | J. RENDERING PROVIDER ID.# |
|---|---|---|---|---|---|---|---|---|---|---|---|---|---|---|
| | From MM DD YY | | | To MM DD YY | | | | | | | | | | |
| 1 | 10 09 2008 | | 10 09 2008 | | | 11 | | 99212 ← Procedure | 1 | 97 00 | 1 | | NPI | |
| 2 | | | | | | | | Linkage | | | | | NPI | |
| 3 | | | | | | | | | | | | | NPI | |
| 4 | | | | | | | | | | | | | NPI | |
| 5 | | | | | | | | | | | | | NPI | |
| 6 | | | | | | | | | | | | | NPI | |

25. FEDERAL TAX I.D. NUMBER   SSN ☐ EIN ☒   **16 1234567**    26. PATIENT'S ACCOUNT NO. **HUANGER0**    27. ACCEPT ASSIGNMENT? (For govt. claims, see back) ☒ YES ☐ NO    28. TOTAL CHARGE $ **97 00**   29. AMOUNT PAID $ **0 00**   30. BALANCE DUE $

31. SIGNATURE OF PHYSICIAN OR SUPPLIER INCLUDING DEGREES OR CREDENTIALS (I certify that the statements on the reverse apply to this bill and are made a part thereof.)
**SIGNATURE ON FILE**
SIGNED _____ DATE _____

32. SERVICE FACILITY LOCATION INFORMATION
**SAME**
a. NPI   b.

33. BILLING PROVIDER INFO & PHONE # ( )
**CHRISTOPHER CONNOLLY MD**
**1400 WEST CENTER ST**
**TOLEDO OH 43601**
NPI **1286927799**   b.

CARRIER ↕
PATIENT AND INSURED INFORMATION ↕
PHYSICIAN OR SUPPLIER INFORMATION ↕

## VALLEY ASSOCIATES, PC
1400 West Center Street
Toledo, OH 43601-0123
614-321-0987

**PATIENT INFORMATION FORM**

| THIS SECTION REFERS TO PATIENT ONLY | | | |
|---|---|---|---|
| **Name:** Shelley Simon | **Sex:** F | **Marital Status:** D ☐S ☐M ☑D ☐W | **Birth Date:** 7/21/52 |
| **Address:** 14 West St. | **SS#:** 000-33-3333 | | |

| | | | | | |
|---|---|---|---|---|---|
| **City:** Toledo | **State:** OH | **Zip:** 43601 | **Employer:** Harmon Bros. | | **Phone:** 555-666-7727 |
| **Home Phone:** 555-111-2222 | | | **Employer's Address:** 18 Bay St. | | |
| **Work Phone:** 555-666-7727 | | | **City:** Toledo | **State:** OH | **Zip:** 43601 |
| **Spouse's Name:** | | | **Spouse's Employer:** | | |
| **Emergency Contact:** Allen King | | | **Relationship:** Brother | **Phone #:** 555-111-7788 | |

| FILL IN IF PATIENT IS A MINOR | | | |
|---|---|---|---|
| **Parent/Guardian's Name:** | **Sex:** | **Marital Status:** ☐S ☐M ☐D ☐W | **Birth Date:** |
| **Phone:** | **SS#:** | | |
| **Address:** | **Employer:** | | **Phone:** |
| **City:** **State:** **Zip:** | **Employer's Address:** | | |
| **Student Status:** | **City:** **State:** **Zip:** | | |

| INSURANCE INFORMATION | |
|---|---|
| **Primary Insurance Company:** Guardian Health | **Secondary Insurance Company:** None |
| **Subscriber's Name:** Patient   **Birth Date:** | **Subscriber's Name:**   **Birth Date:** |
| **Plan:** Superior   **SS#:** 000-33-3333 | **Plan:** |
| **Policy #:** 666000   **Group #:** 7N921 | **Policy #:**   **Group #:** |
| **Copayment/Deductible:**   **Price Code:** | |

| OTHER INFORMATION | |
|---|---|
| **Reason for visit:** Flulike symptoms | **Allergy to Medication (list):** Penicillin |
| **Name of referring physician:** | **If auto accident, list date and state in which it occurred:** |

I authorize treatment and agree to pay all fees and charges for the person named above. I agree to pay all charges shown by statements, promptly upon their presentation, unless credit arrangements are agreed upon in writing.

I authorize payment directly to VALLEY ASSOCIATES, PC of insurance benefits otherwise payable to me. I hereby authorize the release of any medical information necessary in order to process a claim for payment in my behalf.

*Shelley Simon*
_____          _____
(Patient's Signature/Parent or Guardian's Signature)                                    (Date)

I plan to make payment of my medical expenses as follows (check one or more):

_✓_ Insurance (as above)   ____Cash/Check/Credit/Debit Card   ____Medicare   ____Medicaid   ____Workers' Comp.

## Speaking

You will have to speak directly to clients in person or on the phone. You will speak to coworkers, medical practitioners, suppliers, and anyone else who comes in to a medical practice. In all cases, honor everyone's privacy, remember the legal and ethical rules before disclosing any information, speak clearly enough to make sure you are understood, and always be courteous.

**Situation 1:** You are a medical receptionist and Mary Z. has just arrived 30 minutes early for an appointment. She is anxious to know if she can be taken right away. You have to inform her that the doctor is busy but will take her as soon as possible. The waiting room has many magazines as well as a television and there is an interesting news show about to start. Describe how you would handle the situation.

_____

_____

_____

_____

**Situation 2:** You are a phlebotomist in a small laboratory. Justin is 6 years old and is about to have his blood drawn. You explain to him that you are going to put a rubber strap around his arm and that he should make a fist squeezing his fingers together as hard as he can and then you show him the small needle you will insert into his vein. Write briefly describing how you would talk to Justin.

_____

_____

_____

_____

**Situation 3:** You are a billing clerk in a medical office and you have to explain to an elderly patient on the phone that $30 of her bill is not covered by Medicare and that she will have to bring a check in at her upcoming visit. Describe your telephone conversation in which you have her repeat the information so you are sure she understands exactly what she has to do.

_____

_____

_____

_____

## Listening

Health care workers often help patients just by listening and giving words of comfort. You are a nursing assistant in a convalescent home. Many of the patients are elderly who are recovering from broken bones such as broken hips. They are often disoriented and lonely. Part of your job is to help them focus on tasks such as eating. Jim L. is doing fine with his physical therapy but has lost 5 pounds in the last two weeks. The staff dietician has left instructions for his meals to be monitored. You are making sure Jim eats breakfast including two slices of toast, one egg, and a bowl of mixed fruit. Jim seems to do better at eating when someone sits and listens to him. Describe how you would ask him about his family while encouraging him to eat.

_____

_____

_____

_____

## Writing

You are a medical assistant working for a family practitioner. Adele M. is being referred to a neurologist for testing for suspected multiple sclerosis. You are sending a referral letter and her records for an appointment in a week. Complete the following referral letter for this patient.

_____

Robert Blakiston, MD
455 Harley Lane
Handley, Utah 00009

Dear Dr. Blakiston:

This letter is a follow-up to our conversation of Tuesday, May 11. I discussed

_____

_____

_____

_____

Enclosed are _____

_____. To confirm, her appointment

_____.

Thank you for taking this patient.

Sincerely yours,

Elena Simons, MD

# Prefixes

## Prefixes in Medical Terminology

In this unit, you will learn many prefixes that are commonly used in medical terms. When combined with the word parts in Units 4 through 16, you will be able to build many medical terms. In addition, knowing these prefixes will help you understand unfamiliar medical terms.

Some medical prefixes that describe *size* or *quantity* include:

| Prefix | Meaning | Prefix | Meaning |
|---|---|---|---|
| bi- | twice, double | multi- | many |
| brachy- | short | olig(o)- | few, little, scanty |
| hemi- | half | pan-, pant(o)- | all, entire |
| iso- | equal, same | pluri- | several, more |
| meg(a)-, megal(o)- | large | poly- | many |
| micr(o)- | small, microscopic | quadra-, quadri- | four |
| mon(o)- | single | uni- | one |

Some medical prefixes that describe *position* or *location* include:

| Prefix | Meaning | Prefix | Meaning |
|---|---|---|---|
| ab-, abs- | away from | epi- | over |
| ad- | toward, to | ex- | out of, away from |
| ana- | up, toward | exo- | external, on the outside |
| apo- | derived, separate | extra- | without, on the outside |
| cata- | down | infra- | positioned beneath |
| circum- | around | inter- | between |
| di-, dif-, dir-, dis- | not, separated | intra- | within |
| dia- | through | mes(o)- | middle, median |
| ect(o)- | outside | per- | through, intensely |
| end(o)- | within | peri- | around, about, near |

| Prefix | Meaning | Prefix | Meaning |
|--------|---------|--------|---------|
| retro- | behind, backward | supra- | above, over |
| sub- | less than, under, inferior | trans- | across, through |

Some medical prefixes that describe **time** include:

| Prefix | Meaning | Prefix | Meaning |
|--------|---------|--------|---------|
| ante- | before | pre- | before |
| post- | after, following | pro- | before, forward |

Some medical prefixes that describe the **presence** or **quality** of a specific factor that influences the meaning of the word include:

| Prefix | Meaning | Prefix | Meaning |
|--------|---------|--------|---------|
| a- | without | hyper- | above normal, overly, excessive |
| ambi- | both, around | | |
| an- | without | hypo- | below normal, insufficient |
| anti- | against | mal- | bad, inadequate |
| brady- | slow | non- | not, reverse of |
| co-, col-, com-, con-, cor- | together | re- | again, backward |
| | | semi- | half |
| contra- | against | syl-, sym-, syn-, sys- | together |
| de- | away from | tachy- | fast |
| dys- | abnormal, difficult | ultra- | beyond, excessive |
| eu- | well, good, normal | un- | not |

Several miscellaneous medical prefixes include:

| Prefix | Meaning | Prefix | Meaning |
|--------|---------|--------|---------|
| allo- | other, different | par(a)- | beside, abnormal, involving two parts |
| auto- | self | | |
| hetero- | other, different | xeno- | foreign |
| meta- | after | | |

## Building Terms

Add a prefix to complete each of the following terms.

1.  removal of pressure: _____ compression

2.  outside of a cell: _____ cellular

3.  normal thyroid function: _____ thyroid

4.  parasite that lives on the outside: _____ parasite

5.  occurring all around the world: _____ demic

6.  low calcium level in the blood: _____ calcemia

7.  abnormally large head: _____ cephaly

8.  middle of the brain: _____ encephalon

9.  very large heart: _____ cardia

10. away from the mouth: _____ oral

11. outer layer of the heart wall: _____ cardium

12. scalp or cover over the cranium: _____ cranium

13. obsession with one idea: _____ mania

14. difficult menstruation: _____ menorrhea

15. within the heart: _____ cardial

16. outside of the body: _____ corporeal

17. slow breathing: _____ pnea

18. lacking a head: _____ cephalia

19. drug that kills malaria: _____ malarial

20. conditions with abnormally short fingers: _____ dactyly

21. before a disease is found: _____ clinical

22. normal breathing: _____ pnea

23. excessive insulin: _____ insulinism

24. abnormally fast breathing: _____ ventilation

25. scanty menstruation: _____ menorrhea

## Figuring Out the Meaning

Define each of the following terms. The definition of certain word parts are given next to the parts.

1. copayment: _____

2. hyperactive: _____

3. malabsorption: _____

4. postoperative: _____

5. antidepressant: _____

6. noncompliance: _____

7. bradycardia (heart): _____

8. dysfunctional: _____

9. megacolon: _____

10. bilateral (side): _____

11. hypoadrenalism (adrenal activity): _____

12. midbrain: _____

13. postmenopause: _____

14. prediabetic: _____

15. bradykinetic (movement): _____

16. pansinusitis (sinus inflammation): _____

17. monomyoplegia (muscle paralysis): _____

18. contraindicated: _____

19. nonprescription: _____

20. dysphagia (swallowing): _____

21. hyperkinesias (muscular activity): _____

22. multicellular: _____

23. endocervix: _____

24. premature: _____

25. megavitamin: _____

## Using the Dictionary

Choose 20 prefixes from the lists in this unit. Using your allied health dictionary, write down at least two words for each prefix. Break each word down into word parts and write its definition.

1. _____

2. _____

3. _____

4. _____

5. _____

6. _____

7. _____

8. _____

9. _____

10. _____

11. _____

12. _____

13. _____

14. _____

15. _____

16. _____

17. _____

18. _____

19. _____

20. _____

21. _____

22. _____

23. _____

24. _____

25. _____

26. _____

27. _____

28. _____

29. _____

30. _____

31. _____

32. _____

33. _____

34. _____

35. _____

36. _____

37. _____

38. _____

39. _____

40. _____

## Using Flashcards

Using the flashcards bound in with this book, build at least ten medical terms using prefixes and define the terms.

1. _____

2. _____

3. _____

4. _____

5. _____

6. _____

7. _____

8. _____

9. _____

10. _____

# 3

# Suffixes

## Suffixes in Medical Terminology

In this unit, you will learn many suffixes that are commonly used in medical terms. When combined with the word parts in Units 4 through 16, you will be able to build many medical terms. In addition, knowing these suffixes will help you understand unfamiliar medical terms.

Some medical suffixes that describe *sensations* or *feelings* that influence the meaning of the word include:

| Suffix | Meaning | Suffix | Meaning |
|---|---|---|---|
| -algia | pain | -kinisia | movement |
| -asthenia | weakness | -kinesis | movement |
| -desis | binding | -phobia | fear |
| -dynia | pain | -phonia | sound |
| -esthesia | sensation | -phoria | feeling; carrying |

## Conditions/Condition-related

| Suffix | Meaning | Suffix | Meaning |
|---|---|---|---|
| -cele | hernia | -mania | obsession |
| -cytosis | condition of cells | -megaly | enlargement |
| -ectasia | expansion; dilation | -oma (pl. —omata) | tumor, neoplasm |
| -ectasis | expanding; dilating | -opia | vision |
| -edema | swelling | -opsia | vision |
| -ema | condition | -osis (pl. —oses) | condition, state, process |
| -emesis | vomiting | | |
| -iasis | pathological condition or state | -paresis | slight paralysis |
| | | -pathy | disease |
| -ism | condition, disease | -penia | deficiency |
| -itis (pl. —itides) | inflammation | -philia | attraction; affinity for |
| -lepsy | condition of | -phrenia | of the mind |
| -leptic | having seizures | -phthisis | wasting away |

| Suffix | Meaning | Suffix | Meaning |
|--------|---------|--------|---------|
| -physis | growing | -rrhea | discharge |
| -plegia | paralysis | -rrhagia | heavy discharge |
| -plegic | one who is paralyzed | -rrhexis | rupture |
| -ptosis | falling down; drooping | -trophic | nutritional |
| | | -trophy | nutrition |

## Body Parts, Elements, etc.

| Suffix | Meaning | Suffix | Meaning |
|--------|---------|--------|---------|
| -cyte | cell | -globulin | protein |
| -derma | skin | -oxia | oxygen |
| -emia | blood | -plakia | plaque |
| -emic | relating to blood | -plasm | formation |
| -globin | protein | -uria | urine |

## Surgical/Procedural

| Suffix | Meaning | Suffix | Meaning |
|--------|---------|--------|---------|
| -ectomy | removal of | -rrhaphy | surgical suturing |
| -lysis | destruction of | -static | maintaining a state |
| -lytic | destroying | -stomy | opening |
| -ostomy | opening | -tome | cutting instrument, segment |
| -pexy | fixation, usually done surgically | -tomy | cutting operation |
| -plasty | surgical repair | | |

## Pathology/Diagnostic

| Suffix | Meaning | Suffix | Meaning |
|--------|---------|--------|---------|
| -crit | separate | -graph | recording instrument |
| -gen | producing, coming to be | -graphy | process of recording |
| | | -meter | measuring device |
| -genesis | production of | -metry | measurement |
| -genic | producing | -opsy | view of |
| -gram | a recording | -pheresis | removal |

Name _____

Class _____  Date _____

| Suffix | Meaning | Suffix | Meaning |
|--------|---------|--------|---------|
| -phil | attraction, affinity for | -scopy | use of an instrument for observing |
| -scope | instrument (esp. one used for observing or measuring) | | |

## Miscellaneous

| Suffix | Meaning | Suffix | Meaning |
|--------|---------|--------|---------|
| -ad | toward | -oid | like, resembling |
| -clasis | breaking | -phylaxis | protection |
| -clast | breaking instrument | -plegic | one who is paralyzed |
| -form | in the shape of | -stat | agent to maintain a state |
| -ic | pertaining to | | |
| -ics | treatment, practice, body of knowledge | -tropia | turning |
| | | -tropic | turning toward |
| -logist | one who practices | -tropy | condition of turning toward |
| -logy | study, practice | | |
| | | -version | turning |

## Building Terms

Add a suffix to complete each of the following terms.

**1.** practitioner who treats blood disorders: hemato_____

**2.** ear inflammation: ot_____

**3.** breaking of a bone: osteo_____

**4.** unusually heavy menstruation: meno_____

**5.** removal of the appendix: append_____

**6.** kidney disease: reno_____

**7.** heart enlargement: cardio_____

**8.** instrument for observing the intestines: entero_____

**9.** paralysis of half of the body: hemi_____

**10.** bone pain: osteo_____

11. sugar production: gluco_____

12. faulty movement: dys_____

13. lack of oxygen: an_____

14. nose job: rhino_____

15. surgical opening in the colon: colono_____

16. drooping eyelid: blepharo_____

17. hernia in the bladder: cysto_____

18. scanty urination: olig_____

19. muscle tumor: my_____

20. feeling of well-being: eu_____

21. fear of night: nycto_____

22. stomach pain: gastr_____

23. condition with sleep seizures: narco_____

24. a turning backward: retro_____

25. obsession with a single idea: mono_____

## Figuring Out the Meaning

Define each of the following terms. The definition of certain word parts are given next to the parts.

1. cephal(head)ad: _____

2. tars(ankle)ectomy: _____

3. abdomino(abdomen)scopy: _____

4. carcino(cancer)gen: _____

5. rhino(nose)rrhagia: _____

6. bronchi(bronchus)ectasis: _____

7. tendino(tendon)plasty: _____

8. chondro(cartilage)cyte: _____

9. acidosis: _____

10. retino(retina)pathy: _____

11. nyct(night)uria: _____

12. mammo(breast)gram: _____

13. burs(bursa)itis: _____

14. salpingo(fallopian tube)cele: _____

15. uremia: _____

16. colpo(vaginal)dynia: _____

17. angio(blood vessel)rrhaphy: _____

18. bradykinesia: _____

19. cardiorrhexis: _____

20. ceco(cecum)pexy: _____

21. crani(skull)al: _____

22. mast(breast)oid: _____

23. pathology: _____

24. neuro(nerve)cyte: _____

25. sclera(sclera)ectasia: _____

## Using the Dictionary

For each of the body system word parts given, find five words that use suffixes in this unit. Using your allied health dictionary, break the word down into word parts and write its definition.

1. Integumentary system: dermat(o), skin; melan(o), black; lip(o), fat; xer(o), dry.

    a. _____

    b. _____

    c. _____

    d. _____

    e. _____

**2.** Musculoskeletal system: oste(o), bone; my(o), muscle; arthr(o), joint.

a. _____

b. _____

c. _____

d. _____

e. _____

**3.** Cardiovascular system: cardi(o), heart; angi(o), blood vessel; phleb(o), vein; arteri(o), artery.

a. _____

b. _____

c. _____

d. _____

e. _____

**4.** Respiratory system: bronchi(o), bronchus; pneum(o), pneumon(o), lung; alveoli(o), alveolus.

a. _____

b. _____

c. _____

d. _____

e. _____

**5.** Nervous system: cerebr(o), cerebrum; encephal(o), brain; neur(o), nerve; myel(o), spinal cord.

a. _____

b. _____

c. _____

d. _____

e. _____

6. Urinary system: nephr(o), kidney; cyst(o), bladder; ur(o), urine.

    **a.** _____

    **b.** _____

    **c.** _____

    **d.** _____

    **e.** _____

7. Female reproductive system: mast(o), breast; uter(o), uterus; colp(o), vagina.

    **a.** _____

    **b.** _____

    **c.** _____

    **d.** _____

    **e.** _____

8. Male reproductive system: sperm(o), spermat(o), sperm; prostate(o), prostate; orchid(o), testes.

    **a.** _____

    **b.** _____

    **c.** _____

    **d.** _____

    **e.** _____

9. Blood system: hemat(o), blood; erythr(o), red; leuk(o), white.

    **a.** _____

    **b.** _____

    **c.** _____

    **d.** _____

    **e.** _____

10. Lymphatic and immune systems: lymph(o), lymph; immune(o), immunity; tox(o), poison.

   a. _____

   b. _____

   c. _____

   d. _____

   e. _____

11. Digestive system: gastr(o), stomach; enter(o), intestines; col(o), colon(o)-, colon.

   a. _____

   b. _____

   c. _____

   d. _____

   e. _____

12. Endocrine system: aden(o), gland; gluc(o), glucose; thyr(o), thyroid.

   a. _____

   b. _____

   c. _____

   d. _____

   e. _____

13. Sensory system: opthalm(o), eye; ot(o), ear; nas(o), nose.

   a. _____

   b. _____

   c. _____

   d. _____

   e. _____

## Using Flashcards

Using the flashcards bound in with this book, build at least ten medical terms using suffixes and define the terms.

1. _____

2. _____

3. _____

4. _____

5. _____

6. _____

7. _____

8. _____

9. _____

10. _____

# Terms in the Integumentary System

## Word Parts in the Integumentary System

These are the major word parts used to form words in the integumentary system. When you combine these parts with some of the prefixes and suffixes in Units 2 and 3, you will be able to understand medical terms relating to the integumentary system.

| | |
|---|---|
| adip(o) | fatty |
| dermat(o) | skin |
| derm(o), -derma | skin |
| hidr(o) | sweat, sweat glands |
| ichthy(o) | fish, scaly |
| kerat(o) | horny tissue |
| lip(o) | fatty |
| melan(o) | black, very dark |
| myc(o) | fungus |
| onych(o) | nail |
| pil(o) | hair |
| seb(o) | sebum, sebaceous glands |
| steat(o) | fat |
| trich(o) | hair |
| xanth(o) | yellow |
| xer(o) | dry |

After practicing word building and terminology exercises related to the integumentary system, you will follow a patient with a skin problem through diagnosis and treatment.

# Exercises in the Integumentary System

## Building Terms

For each of the following definitions, provide a term using integumentary system word parts as well as prefixes and suffixes you learned in Units 2 and 3.

1. plastic surgery using skin grafts: _____

2. skin rash caused by a fungus: _____

3. hairlike: _____

4. condition with fatty deposits in tissue: _____

5. fat cell: _____

6. fungal infection of the nail: _____

7. fatty tumor (give 3 terms): _____, _____, _____

8. dry skin: _____

9. condition with excessive pigment in the skin: _____

10. disease or condition caused by a fungus: _____

## Completing Terms

Complete the following terms by adding a prefix or suffix to the word or word part given here.

1. pigmented cell: melano_____

2. beneath the skin: _____cutaneous

3. without pigmentation: _____pigmentation

4. yellowish growth or tumor: xanth_____

5. skin inflammation: dermat_____

6. into the skin: _____dermal

7. foreign skin graft (as from an animal): _____ graft

8. practice of integumentary medicine: dermato_____

9. below the skin (as a needle): _____dermic

10. anti-itch agent: _____pruritic

## Finding the Word Parts

Break each of the following terms into words or word parts. Give the definition of the term as well as the meaning of each word or word part.

1.  melanoderma: _____

    _____

2.  trichoid: _____

    _____

3.  dermoplasty: _____

    _____

4.  xanthoderma: _____

    _____

5.  keratosis: _____

    _____

6.  seborrhea: _____

    _____

7.  ichthyosis: _____

    _____

8.  adipocyte: _____

    _____

9.  hidrosis: _____

    _____

10. steatorrhea: _____

    _____

11. allograft: _____

    _____

12. autograft: _____

    _____

**13.** xenograft: _____

_____

**14.** intradermal: _____

_____

**15.** lipoma: _____

_____

## Proofreading and Understanding Terms

Write the correct spelling and definition in the blank to the right of any misspelled words. If the spelling is correct, write C.

**1.** suderiferus: _____

**2.** integument: _____

**3.** alopesia: _____

**4.** papule: _____

**5.** cicatriz: _____

**6.** vitilligo: _____

**7.** scleroderma: _____

**8.** celullitis: _____

**9.** epithileum: _____

**10.** psoriasis: _____

**11.** neoplasm: _____

**12.** dicubitus ulcer: _____

**13.** dabridement: _____

**14.** carbuncle: _____

**15.** excisional biopsy: _____

In the following referral letter, find at least 5 misspellings and correct them.

**Dr. Samuel Cherkin**
732 Swann Street
Rochester, NY 99999

Dear Dr. Cherkin:

This letter is to conform the referral of Susan Ayles to your office. Ms. Ayles is a new patient who has an intractable case of porsiasis. She just moved here from California and has never seen a dermatologist, having dealt with the problem using over-the-counter medication. She says that it has worsend recently. Mr. Ayles is 25-years-old and is an emmployee of the university. Her first appointment with me was for a fysical. I am enclosing a copy of her CDC (complete blood count) for your records.

Please send a report to me once you have examined the patient and set a cors of treatment.

Sincerely yours,

*Ellen Larsen, MD*

Ellen Larsen, MD

_____

_____

_____

_____

_____

_____

_____

_____

## Fill in the Blanks

1. Bx is the abbreviation for _____.

2. The lunula appears at the base of the _____.

3. Surgery to remove excess adipose tissue is _____.

4. A(n) _____ is a skin graft from one's own body.

5. Excessive hairiness is called _____.

6. The medical term for a blackhead is _____.

7. Malignant _____ is a potentially fatal type of skin cancer.

8. Lice infestation is _____.

9. Another name for a wart is _____.

10. A cold sore is a type of Herpes simplex type _____ virus.

11. Chickenpox can remain dormant and show up later in life as _____.

12. The rule of nines is a method of categorizing _____.

13. The use of _____ can help avoid skin cancer.

14. Removal of a plug of skin for examination is called a(n) _____.

15. A reaction to physical contact with an allergen is called _____ dermatitis.

## True or False

Circle T for true or F for false.

1. Tinea pedis occurs in the hair.     T   F

2. An allograft uses the patient's own skin.     T   F

3. Benign growths are not cancerous.     T   F

4. Melanin is excessive in albinism.     T   F

5. A hematoma always appears subcutaneously.     T   F

6. Petechia are pinpoint hemorrhages in the skin.     T   F

7. Epithelial tissue only appears inside bone.     T   F

8. Sebaceous glands are a type of endocrine gland.   T   F

9. The outermost layer of skin is the epidermis.   T   F

10. Alopecia only occurs in men.   T   F

11. Eczema is a type of cancerous lesion.   T   F

12. Hives can be caused by an allergy.   T   F

13. The dermis is above the epidermis.   T   F

14. A birthmark is also known as a pustule.   T   F

15. Gangrene is contagious.   T   F

## Write the Medical Term

For each of the following descriptions, write the proper medical term.

1. itchy rash: _____

2. nail disease: _____

3. skin disease: _____

4. fatty tumor: _____

5. fungal condition: _____

6. loss of hair; baldness: _____

7. dry skin: _____

8. teenage pimples: _____

9. anti-itch cream: _____

10. skin doctor: _____

11. stitch: _____

12. head lice: _____

13. wart: _____

14. athlete's foot: _____

15. sweat glands: _____

16. birthmark: _____

17. hives: _____

18. cold sore: _____

19. bed sore _____

20. age spot _____

Name _____

Class _____ Date _____

## Word Find

In the following puzzle, draw a line around at least 20 words pertaining to the integumentary system. The words can be horizontal, vertical, diagonal, or upside-down. Write the words on the rules provided. If you do not know the meaning of a word, look it up in your allied health dictionary and make a flash card for future review.

```
s  e  v  b  g  d  a  y  j  u  a  c  h  t  h  y  i  k  l  e
o  p  n  y  a  w  c  n  f  u  r  u  n  c  l  e  m  k  l  a
e  d  v  a  a  q  n  t  y  h  f  e  x  d  g  h  r  y  r  i
j  k  m  n  r  w  e  w  r  t  g  v  b  n  m  k  e  p  q  r
d  o  d  m  k  u  q  b  n  n  y  j  h  f  d  s  c  v  e  t
a  q  e  r  y  h  p  o  i  p  l  o  j  u  g  h  t  d  m  s
e  n  r  o  c  q  s  r  x  c  v  b  l  e  s  i  o  n  q  y
h  o  m  e  y  b  t  m  u  k  u  t  r  x  a  e  g  h  j  r
e  y  a  n  o  s  t  l  o  p  x  o  t  y  i  k  l  o  p  i
t  o  t  y  a  a  g  h  m  k  s  o  s  i  m  r  e  d  o  n
i  x  i  n  k  l  w  q  o  d  o  e  m  k  l  o  p  a  q  g
h  h  t  u  r  p  l  e  l  m  q  u  b  l  y  n  k  e  l  w
w  z  i  v  g  e  h  o  t  k  l  o  p  u  m  a  e  h  q  o
j  k  s  v  t  v  c  q  g  t  e  c  r  v  m  n  m  k  w  r
q  j  k  b  e  v  q  l  n  r  o  l  o  p  n  c  y  c  l  m
z  x  y  e  u  s  m  k  u  o  a  p  m  a  y  q  m  a  t  k
y  h  f  b  c  q  e  s  z  e  a  f  u  s  c  h  i  l  f  m
e  r  o  p  o  s  k  h  q  a  c  t  b  i  o  m  b  a  k
q  w  x  c  d  i  r  w  k  l  i  s  o  p  c  r  v  q  r  g
k  i  o  p  f  l  y  u  o  p  l  y  i  v  o  n  m  w  g  q
c  a  l  b  i  n  i  s  m  v  n  y  k  s  i  o  l  p  n  b
q  m  n  j  k  m  l  y  h  e  k  l  a  o  o  p  l  c  i  v
e  e  r  b  y  d  n  j  u  z  i  c  o  t  k  t  o  p  k  c
e  z  q  u  k  i  l  q  o  p  e  v  c  w  s  q  a  e  s  i
l  c  p  e  q  o  a  n  k  a  o  p  x  n  j  u  w  r  y  i
a  e  y        l  l  x  c  e  t  u  i  o  l  p  b  r  c  e  q
a  t  g  h  p  e  j  o  p  n  a  m  s  a  o  l  h  c  z  k
h  k  l        o  k  o  t  i  n  e  a  l  p  f  n  y  r  d  a
```

a. _____       n. _____

b. _____       o. _____

c. _____       p. _____

d. _____       q. _____

e. _____       r. _____

f. _____       s. _____

g. _____       t. _____

h. _____       u. _____

i. _____       v. _____

j. _____       w. _____

k. _____       x. _____

l. _____       y. _____

m. _____       z. _____

## Find the Meaning

In the following referral letter, find the terms in the integumentary system. Define them.

---

**Dr. Alicia Williams**
45 Essex Street
Anywhere, TX 99999

Dear Dr. Jones,

In the near future, you will be seeing a patient of mine, Lee Hong. He has been seen by me several times for treatment of verruca on his hands. They have been resistant to liquid nitrogen treatment.

On examination of his hands, there is an approximate 3-mm growth over the dorsum of the index finger and a small lesion on the thumb of his right hand. In addition, I noticed a change in a mole on his left thigh. Please check this mole.

Thank you for assisting in the care of this patient.

Sincerely,

*Alicia Williams*

Alicia Williams, MD

---

_____

_____

_____

_____

_____

_____

_____

_____

## Follow the Patient

The exercises that follow will take you through a patient case study for this unit. The patient is Melissa Sterron. She lives at 425 Oakland Drive, Sand Hill, MD 00022.

## Fill in the Blanks

Melissa Sterron has had an itchy rash (pruritus) on her arm for about a week. This is the third time this rash has appeared. She called her primary physician who suggested it was time to see a specialist so her doctor provided a referral letter to a _____. This specialist will be able to take a shave biopsy of the rash to determine the cause. It could be a _____ (fungal condition) or just reoccurring _____ (dryness).

## Make the Patient Call

The medical assistant, Andrew Weston, first asks Melissa the following information and, while he is talking to her on the phone, fills in the call memo below.

1. He confirms that her insurance is still the same and he repeats the name of her plan: Blue Stream Health Care, subscriber number 3456787.
2. He asks her what days of the week she will be available and what hours are best: Melissa is off on Tuesdays and Thursdays and any time of the day is fine.
3. He tells Melissa that the specialist's office will send her a confirmation letter with medical history forms for her to complete and bring to her visit.

## Complete the Phone Call Form

Fill in the missing information on the phone call slip.

Date_____ Time of Call_____ am___ pm___

Name_____

Phone_____

Message_____

_____

_____

Best time to call _____ E-mail_____

## Call the Specialist

Next, Andrew calls Dr. Manganara's office to schedule a referral appointment for Melissa Sterron.

Fill in the missing information.

Good morning, this is Andrew Weston from Dr. Allen's office. I need to refer a patient to Dr. Manganara. Her name is _____. Her insurance is _____ and she is available on _____ and _____ all day.

Theresa Martin, the receptionist in Dr. Manganara's office makes the appointment for Thursday, January 5 at 3:00. Dr. Manganara uses a computer for scheduling as well as a backup written system.

Enter the information for Melissa's appointment into the scheduling book.

Scheduler
January

| Time | Monday | Tuesday | Wednesday | Thursday | Friday | Saturday |
|------|--------|---------|-----------|----------|--------|----------|
| 9:00-9:15 | | | | | | |
| 9:15-9:30 | | | | | | |
| 9:30-9:45 | | | | | | |
| 9:45-10:00 | | | | | | |
| 10:00-10:15 | | | | | | |
| 10:15-10:30 | | | | | | |
| 10:30-10:45 | | | | | | |
| 10:45-11:00 | | | | | | |
| 11:15-11:30 | | | | | | |
| 11:30-11:45 | | | | | | |
| 11:45-12:00 | | | | | | |
| 12:00-1:30 | xxxxx | xxxxx | xxxxxx | xxxxx | xxxxx | xxxxx |
| 1:30-1:45 | | | | | | |
| 1:45-2:00 | | | | | | |
| 2:00-2:15 | | | | | | |
| 2:15-2:30 | | | | | | |
| 2:30-2:45 | | | | | | |
| 2:45-3:00 | | | | | | |
| 3:00-3:15 | | | | | | |
| 3:15-3:30 | | | | | | |
| 3:30-3:45 | | | | | | |
| 3:45-4:00 | | | | | | |
| 4:00-4:15 | | | | | | |
| 4:15-4:30 | | | | | | |
| 4:30-4:45 | | | | | | |
| 4:45-5:00 | | | | | | |
| 5:00-5:15 | | | | | | |
| 5:15-5:30 | | | | | | |
| 5:30-5:45 | | | | | | |
| 5:45-6:00 | | | | | | |

Next, write the letter that Theresa will send to Melissa. Make sure to ask her to arrive 15 minutes early so paperwork can be checked and completed. What form does she need to include? _____.

**Dr. James Manganara**
777 Reston Street
Anywhere, US 99999


Dear _____ :

_____

_____

_____

_____

_____

_____

_____

_____

_____

_____

## The Appointment

The day before the appointment, Theresa places a call to Melissa. She is not at home. Theresa leaves the following message on her answering machine.

Hello Melissa, this is Dr. Manganara's office. You have an appointment tomorrow, Thursday,

January 5 at _____. Please arrive at _____ and make sure to

bring the completed _____ and your insurance card.

Melissa arrives on time. She hands in her form and gives Theresa her insurance card. Theresa xeroxes the card and puts the medical history form in a new folder. She gives Melissa a patient information form, privacy and confidentiality information form, and a payment form.

## Handling the Paperwork

Theresa has to check the paperwork to make sure it is completed correctly.

Fill in the missing information on the form on page 46.

Dr. Manganara examines Melissa's rash and believes it to be fungal. To be certain, he takes a scraping to be sent to the laboratory for culturing. He says that he will call her with the results and will prescribe an ointment to be used for 10 days if it is fungal.

Fill out the laboratory form on page 49.

A follow-up appointment is scheduled and Theresa gives the folder to Amy, the billing clerk. Amy gives Melissa a receipt and submits the insurance electronically.

A paper bill is also prepared. Fill in the information on the paper form shown on page 48.

## Dr. James Manganara
777 Reston Street
Anywhere, US 99999
555-555-5555

**PATIENT INFORMATION FORM**

### THIS SECTION REFERS TO PATIENT ONLY

| Name:  Melissa Sterron | Sex: F | Marital Status: D  ☐S ☐M ☐D ☐W | Birth Date: 7/21/52 |
|---|---|---|---|

| Address: | SS#:  000-33-3333 |
|---|---|

| City: | State: OH | Zip: | Employer: | Phone: |
|---|---|---|---|---|

| Home Phone: | Employer's Address: |
|---|---|

| Work Phone: | City: | State: | Zip: |
|---|---|---|---|

| Spouse's Name: | Spouse's Employer: |
|---|---|

| Emergency Contact: | Relationship: | Phone #: |
|---|---|---|

### FILL IN IF PATIENT IS A MINOR

| Parent/Guardian's Name: | Sex: | Marital Status:  ☐S ☐M ☐D ☐W | Birth Date: |
|---|---|---|---|

| Phone: | SS#: |
|---|---|

| Address: | Employer: | Phone: |
|---|---|---|

| City: | State: | Zip: | Employer's Address: |
|---|---|---|---|

| Student Status: | City: | State: | Zip: |
|---|---|---|---|

### INSURANCE INFORMATION

| Primary Insurance Company: | Secondary Insurance Company: None |
|---|---|

| Subscriber's Name: | Birth Date: | Subscriber's Name: | Birth Date: |
|---|---|---|---|

| Plan: | SS#: | Plan: |
|---|---|---|

| Policy #: | Group #: | Policy #: | Group #: |
|---|---|---|---|

| Copayment/Deductible: | Price Code: | |
|---|---|---|

### OTHER INFORMATION

| Reason for visit: | Allergy to Medication (list): |
|---|---|

| Name of referring physician: | If auto accident, list date and state in which it occurred: |
|---|---|

I authorize treatment and agree to pay all fees and charges for the person named above. I agree to pay all charges shown by statements, promptly upon their presentation, unless credit arrangements are agreed upon in writing.

I authorize payment directly to Dr. Manganaro of insurance benefits otherwise payable to me. I hereby authorize the release of any medical information necessary in order to process a claim for payment in my behalf.

_____     _____
(Patient's Signature/Parent or Guardian's Signature)                    (Date)

I plan to make payment of my medical expenses as follows (check one or more):

_✓_ Insurance (as above)  _____ Cash/Check/Credit/Debit Card  _____ Medicare  _____ Medicaid  _____ Workers' Comp.

Name _____

Class _____ Date _____

---

Dr. James Mangonara
777 Reston St.
Anywhere, USA 99999
555-555-5555

☐ PRIVATE ☐ BLUECROSS ☐ IND. ☐ MEDICARE ☐ MEDICAID ☐ HMO ☐ PPO

| PATIENT'S LAST NAME | | FIRST | ACCOUNT # | BIRTHDATE / / | SEX ☐ MALE ☐ FEMALE | TODAY'S DATE / / |
|---|---|---|---|---|---|---|
| INSURANCE COMPANY | | SUBSCRIBER | | PLAN # | SUB. # | GROUP # |

ASSIGNMENT: I hereby assign my insurance benefits to be paid directly to the undersigned physician. I am financially responsible for non-covered services.
SIGNED: (Patient)
Parent (if Minor)                    DATE:    /    /

RELEASE: I hereby authorize the physician to release to my insurance carriers any information requested to process this claim.
SIGNED: (Patient)
Parent (if Minor)                    DATE:    /    /

| ✓ | DESCRIPTION | CPT/Med | Dx/Re | PEE | ✓ | DESCRIPTION | CPT/Med | Dx/Re | PEE | ✓ | DESCRIPTION | CPT/Med | Dx/Re | PEE |
|---|---|---|---|---|---|---|---|---|---|---|---|---|---|---|
| | OFFICE CARE | | | | | PROCEDURES | | | | | INJECTIONS/IMMUNIZATIONS | | | |
| | NEW PATIENT | | | | | Treadmill (in Office) | 93015 | | | | Tetanus | | 90718 | |
| | Brief | 99201 | | | | 24-hour Holter | 93224 | | | | Hypertet | J1870 | 90782 | |
| | Limited | 99202 | | | | if Medicare set-up fee | 93225 | | | | Pneumococcal | | 90732 | |
| | Intermediate | 99203 | | | | Physician Interpret | 93227 | | | | Influenza | | 90724 | |
| | Extended | 99204 | | | | EKG w/Interpretation | 93000 | | | | TB Skin Test (PPD) | | 86585 | |
| | Comprehensive | 99205 | | | | EKG (Medicare) | 93005 | | | | Antigen Injection-Single | | 95115 | |
| | | | | | | Sigmoidoscopy | 45300 | | | | Multiple | | 95117 | |
| | ESTABLISHED PATIENT | | | | | Sigmoidoscopy (flexible) | 45330 | | | | B12 Injection | J3420 | 90782 | |
| | Minimal | 99211 | | | | Sigmoidos., Flex. w/Bx. | 45331 | | | | Injection, IM | | 90782 | |
| | Brief | 99212 | | | | Spirometry FEV/FVC | 94010 | | | | Compazine | J0780 | 90782 | |
| | Limited | 99213 | | | | Spirometry, Post-Dilator | 94080 | | | | Demerol | J2175 | 90782 | |
| | Intermediate | 99214 | | | | | | | | | Vistaril | J3410 | 90782 | |
| | Extended | 99215 | | | | | | | | | Susphrine | J0170 | 90782 | |
| | Comprehensive | 00215 | | | | LABORATORY | | | | | Decadron | J0890 | 90782 | |
| | | | | | | Blood Draw Fee | 36415 | | | | Estradiol | J1000 | 90782 | |
| | CONSULTATION-OFFICE | | | | | Urinalysis, chemical | 81005 | | | | Testosterone | J1080 | 90782 | |
| | Focused | 99241 | | | | Throat Culture | 87081 | | | | Lidocaine | J2000 | 90782 | |
| | Expanded | 99242 | | | | Occult Blood | 82270 | | | | Solumedrol | J2920 | 90782 | |
| | Detailed | 99243 | | | | Pap Handling Charge | 99000 | | | | Solucortel | J1720 | 90782 | |
| | Comprehensive 1 | 99244 | | | | Pap Life Guard | 88150-90 | | | | Hydeltra | J1680 | 90782 | |
| | Comprehensive 2 | 99245 | | | | Gram Stain | 87205 | | | | Oeb Oricaube | H2510 | 90788 | |
| | | | | | | Hanging Drop | 87210 | | | | | | | |
| | | | | | | Urine Drug Screen | 99000 | | | | INJECTIONS-JOINT/BURSA | | | |
| | | | | | | | | | | | Small Joints | | 20800 | |
| | | | | | | | | | | | Intermediate | | 20605 | |
| | | | | | | SUPPLIES | | | | | Large Joints | | 20810 | |
| | | | | | | | | | | | Trigger Point | | 20550 | |
| | | | | | | | | | | | MISCELLANEOUS | | | |

DIAGNOSIS: (ICD-9)

| | | | | | | | | | |
|---|---|---|---|---|---|---|---|---|---|
| __ Abdominal Pain | 789.0 | __ Gout | 274.0 | __ C.V.A. -Acute | 436. | __ Electrolyte Dis. | 276.9 | __ Herpes Simplex | 054.9 |
| __ Abscess (Site) | 682.9 | __ Asthma | 493.90 | __ Cere. Vas. Accid. (Old) | 438 | __ Fatigue | 780.7 | __ Herpes Zoster | 053.9 |
| __ Adverse Drug Rx | 995.2 | __ Asthmatic Bronchitis | 493.90 | __ Cerumen | 380.4 | __ Fibrocys. Br. Dis. | 610.1 | __ Hydrocele | 603.9 |
| __ Alcohol Detox | 291.8 | __ Atrial Fib | 427.31 | __ Chestwall Pain | 786.59 | __ Fracture (Site) | 829.0 | __ Hyperlipidemia | 272.4 |
| __ Alcoholism | 303.90 | __ Atrial Tachi | 427.0 | __ Cholecystitis | 575.0 | __ Open/Close | | __ Hypertension | 401.9 |
| __ Allergic Rhinitis | 477 | __ Bowel Obstruct. | 560.9 | __ Cholelithiasis | 574.00 | __ Fungal Infect. (Site) | 110.8 | __ Hyperthyroidism | 242.9 |
| __ Allergy | 995.3 | __ Breast Mass | 611.72 | __ COPD | 492.8 | __ Gastric Ulcer | 531.90 | __ Hypothyroidism | 244.9 |
| __ Alzheimer's Dis. | 290.1 | __ Bronchitis | 490 | __ Cirrhosis | 571.5 | __ Gastritis | 535.0 | __ Labyrinthitis | 386.30 |
| __ Anemia | 285.9 | __ Bursitis | 727.3 | __ Cong. Heart Fail. | 428.9 | __ Gastroenteritis | 558.9 | __ Lipoma (Site) | 214.9 |
| __ Anemia-Pernicious | 281.0 | __ Cancer, Breast (Site) | 174.9 | __ Conjunctivitis | 372.30 | __ G.I. Bleeding | 578.9 | __ Lymphoma | 202.8 |
| __ Angina | 413.9 | __ Metastatic (Site) | 199.1 | __ Contusion (Site) | 924.9 | __ Glomerulonephritis | 583.9 | __ Mit. Valve Prolapse | 424.0 |
| __ Anxiety Synd. | 300.00 | __ Colon | 153.9 | __ Costochondritis | 733.99 | __ Headache | 784.0 | __ Myocard. Infarction (Area) | 410.9 |
| __ Appendicitis | 541 | __ Cancer, Rectal | 154.1 | __ Depression | 311. | __ Headache, Tension | 307.81 | __ M.I., Old | 412 |
| __ Arterioscl. H.D. | 414.0 | __ Lung (Site) | 162.9 | __ Dermatitis | 692.9 | __ Migrane (Type) | 346.9 | __ Myositis | 729.1 |
| __ Arthritis, Osteo. | 715.90 | __ Skin (Site) | 173.9 | __ Diabetes Mellitus | 250.00 | __ Hemorrhoids | 455.6 | __ Nausea/Vomiting | 767.0 |
| __ Rheumatoid | 714.0 | __ Card. Arrhythmia (Type) | 427.9 | __ Diabetic Ketosis | 250.1 | __ Hernia, Hiatal | 553.3 | __ Neuralgia | 729.2 |
| __ Lupus | 710.0 | __ Cardiomyopathy | 425.4 | __ Diverticulitis | 562.11 | __ Inguinal | 550.9 | __ Nevus (Site) | 216.9 |
| | | __ Cellulitis (Site) | 682.9 | __ Diverticulosis | 562.10 | __ Hepatitis | 573.3 | __ Obesity | 278.0 |

DIAGNOSIS: (IF NOT CHECKED ABOVE)

| SERVICES PERFORMED AT: ☐ Office ☐ E.R. ☐ ☐ CLAIM CONTAINS NO ORDERED REFERRING SERVICE | REFERRING PHYSICIAN & I.D. NUMBER |
|---|---|

| RETURN APPOINTMENT INFORMATION: 5 - 10 - 15 - 20 - 30 - 40 - 60  [ DAYS] [ WKS.] [ MOS.] [ PRN] | NEXT APPOINTMENT M - T - W - TH - F - S DATE / / TIME: | AM PM | ACCEPT ASSIGNMENT? ☐ YES ☐ NO | DOCTOR'S SIGNATURE |
|---|---|---|---|---|

| | ☐ CASH | TOTAL TODAY'S FEE | |
|---|---|---|---|
| 1. Complete upper portion of this form, sign and date. | ☐ CHECK # | OLD BALANCE | |
| 2. Attach this form to your own Insurance company's form for client reimbursement. | | TOTAL DUE | |
| MEDICARE PATIENTS - DO NOT SEND THIS TO MEDICARE. WE WILL SUBMIT THE CLAIM FOR YOU. | ☐ VISA ☐ MC ☐ CO-PAY | AMOUNT REC'D. TODAY | |

# Lab Results

At the laboratory, Steven Melango processed the scraping and filled out the following form.

| FAC CODE | DATE | TIME COLLECTED | LABORATORY USE ONLY |
|---|---|---|---|
| | | : AM | |
| DRAWN BY | | : PM | |

**Archway Diagnostics**
75 Main Street

| CLIENT | PATIENT INFORMATION |
|---|---|

NAME (LAST, FIRST, MIDDLE, INITIAL) — PATIENT ID NO.

ADDRESS

CITY — STATE — ZIPCODE — MALE ☐ FEMALE ☐ DATE OF BIRTH

**ICD CODE (REQUIRED)** — **SYSMPTOM** — PATIENT TELEPHONE NO

PHYSICIAN IF DIFFERENT/REPORTING REMARKS — ☐ FASTING ☐ NON-FASTING

PLEASE BILL TO: ☐ PATIENT BILL ☐ CLIENT/DOCTOR ☐ INSURANCE

REPORTING COMMENTS:

**PRIMARY INSURANCE**

INSURANCE NAME — STATE — INSURED'S NAME

CARBON COPY TO:
(CLIENT CODE OR FULL NAME AND FULL ADDRESS w. ZIP CODE)

RELATIONSHIP TO PATIENT — PATIENT'S (OR INSURED'S) I.D. NUMBER
☐ SELF ☐ SPOUSE ☐ CHILD ☐ OTHER

GROUP NO. — INSURED'S EMPLOYER — PAYOR NUMBER

**SECONDARY INSURANCE**

INSURANCE NAME — STATE — INSURED'S NAME

☐ STAT & CALL — TELEPHONE NUMBER ( )
☐ CALL RESULT — FAX NUMBER ( )
☐ FAX

RELATIONSHIP TO PATIENT — PATIENT'S (OR INSURED'S) I.D. NUMBER
☐ SELF ☐ SPOUSE ☐ CHILD ☐ OTHER

GROUP NO. — INSURED'S EMPLOYER — PAYOR NUMBER

URINE COLLECTION VOLUME — ☐ 24 HOURS ☐ RANDOM
_____ ML: ☐ _____ HRS:

I authorize Archway Diagnostics to release information received, including without limitation, medical information, which includes laboratory test results to my health plan/insurance carrier, and its authorized representatives, I further authorize my health plan/insurance carrier to directly pay Quest Diagnostics for the service rendered.

PATIENT SIGNATURE :

TECHNICAL NOTES:

| LABORATORY USE ONLY 98242 | BLOOD DRAWING FEE 98245 | HANDLING 98253 | HOUSE CALL-PVT 98371 | SINGLE PATIENT-NH 98372 | MULTI PATIENT-NH |
|---|---|---|---|---|---|

| CHEMISTRY TESTS | PANELS/PROFILES | OTHER TESTS | OTHER TESTS |
|---|---|---|---|
| X1234 ☐ Albumin | 226 ☐ Electrolyte Panel | 5647 ☐ Amylase | 4111 ☐ Lyme screen |
| X1233 ☐ Alkaline phosph. | 777 ☐ Lipid Panel | 4333 ☐ Blood group and Rh | 6665 ☐ Progesterone |
| X1245 ☐ ALT (SGPT) | 888 ☐ Metabolic Panel | 6767 ☐ CA-125 | 7676 ☐ Prothrombin time |
| V1222 ☐ AST (SGOT) | 666 ☐ Lipid Panel | 8888 ☐ C-Reactive protein | 8111 ☐ PSA |
| V1234 ☐ Bilirubin, Total | **PROFILES** | 5555 ☐ CBC | 9988 ☐ Testosterone |
| Y3333 ☐ Calcium | 456 ☐ Hepatitis Profiles | 5555A ☐ CBC w/diff | 7676 ☐ Urinalysis complete |
| Y1234 ☐ Carbon Dioxide | 998 ☐ Obstetric Panel | 6789 ☐ Digoxin | 8866 ☐ Vit B12 |
| Y4354 ☐ Chloride | **MICROBIOLOGY** | 7890 ☐ Dilantin | |
| M5555 ☐ Cholesterol | 009 ☐ Chlamydia | 6543 ☐ Estradiol | |
| P6666 ☐ Creatinine | 437 ☐ Gonorrhea | 7776 ☐ Folate | |
| M0099 ☐ Glucose | **Cultures:** | 1221 ☐ FSH | |
| L6565 ☐ Iron | 990 ☐ Blood | 1117 ☐ H. Pylori | |
| Y7777 ☐ Magnesium | 888 ☐ Ear | 2223 ☐ HCG | |
| P0000 ☐ Phosphorus | 777 ☐ Eye | 5556 ☐ HDL | |
| Y3456 ☐ Protein, total | 444 ☐ Genital | 7778 ☐ HIV–W. blot | |
| U7890 ☐ Sodium | 333 ☐ Sputum | 8885 ☐ Herpes | |
| W2345 ☐ Triglycerides | 787 ☐ Stool | 3334 ☐ Iron | |
| Z3456 ☐ Urea nitrogen | | 6667 ☐ Lead | |
| H5555 ☐ Uric acid | | 8787 ☐ LH & FSH | |

Source:
OTHER TESTS:

AUTHORISING PHYSICIAN SIGNATURE

Pick out 5 medical terms from the lab form that relate specifically to the integumentary system and define them in terms that would be easy for the average patient to understand.

_____

_____

_____

_____

_____

## Follow-Up

Dr. Manganara calls Melissa to confirm that the rash is fungal. He says that if the prescription works in 10 days, no follow-up will be needed. He tells her that he will call in a prescription to her pharmacy and transfers her to Theresa to have Melissa give Theresa the information. Theresa takes down the pharmacy information and tells Melissa that she will call it in today. She calls the pharmacy and makes sure to say the full words and no abbreviations according to what she had learned earlier about medical errors. She then asks the pharmacy tech to read back the prescription.

Theresa files Melissa's folder and adds the final diagnosis to Melissa's computer file.

# Terms in the Musculoskeletal System

## Word Parts in the Musculoskeletal System

These are the major word parts used to form words in the musculoskeletal system. When you combine these parts with some of the prefixes and suffixes in Units 2 and 3, you will be able to understand medical terms relating to the musculoskeletal system.

| | |
|---|---|
| acetabul(o) | acetabulum |
| acromi(o) | end point of the scapula |
| ankyl(o) | bent, crooked |
| arthr(o) | joint |
| brachi(o) | arm |
| burs(o) | bursa |
| calcane(o) | heel |
| calci(o) | calcium |
| carp(o) | wrist |
| cephal(o) | head |
| cervic(o) | neck |
| chondr(o) | cartilage |
| condyl(o) | knob, knuckle |
| cost(o) | rib |
| crani(o) | skull |
| dactyl(o) | fingers, toes |
| fasci(o) | fascia |
| femor(o) | femur |
| fibr(o) | fiber |
| humer(o) | humerus |
| ili(o) | ilium |

| | |
|---|---|
| ischi(o) | ischium |
| kyph(o) | hump; bent |
| lamin(o) | lamina |
| leiomy(o) | smooth muscle |
| lumb(o) | lumbar |
| maxill(o) | upper jaw |
| metacarp(o) | metacarpal |
| my(o) | muscle |
| myel(o) | spinal cord; bone marrow |
| oste(o) | bone |
| patell(o) | kneecap |
| ped(i), ped(o) | foot |
| pelv(i) | pelvis |
| phalang(o) | finger or toe bone |
| pod(o) | foot |
| pub(o) | pubis |
| rachi(o) | spine |
| radi(o) | forearm bone |
| rhabd(o) | rod-shaped |
| rhabdomy(o) | striated muscle |
| scapul(o) | scapula |
| scoli(o) | curved |
| spondyl(o) | vertebra |
| stern(o) | sternum |
| synov(o) | synovial membrane |
| tars(o) | tarsus |
| ten(o), tend(o), tendin(o) | tendon |
| thorac(o) | thorax |
| tibi(o) | tibia |
| uln(o) | ulna |
| vertebr(o) | vertebra |

After practicing word building and terminology exercises related to the musculoskeletal system, you will follow a patient with a sports injury who tries to get help through conventional treatment as well as through complementary and alternative medicine.

## Exercises in the Musculoskeletal System

### Building Terms

For each of the following definitions, provide a term using musculoskeletal system word parts as well as prefixes and suffixes you learned in Units 2 and 3.

1. bone tumor: _____

2. inflammation of a vertebra: _____

3. joint pain: _____

4. spinal curvature condition: _____

5. puncture of a joint: _____

6. of or between vertebrae: _____

7. of the arm and the head: _____

8. muscle pain: _____

9. neck inflammation: _____

10. tendon inflammation: _____

11. specialist in foot disorders: _____

12. surgical incision into fibrous tissue: _____

13. of or relating to the thigh: _____

14. plastic surgery on the space at the top of the hipbone:_____

15. fused condition as of a joint: _____

16. device for measuring the pelvis: _____

17. removal of a finger or toe: _____

18. chest pain: _____

19. bone softening: _____

20. tumor with both fibrous and muscle tissue: _____

### Completing Terms

Complete the following terms by adding a prefix or suffix to the word or word part given here.

1. pain in many muscle groups: _____myalgia

2. chest puncture to remove fluid or gas: thoraco_____

3. bone and muscle inflammation: osteomyel_____

4. (injection) into a muscle: _____muscular

5. measurement of the bones of the skull: cranio_____

6. surgical examination of a joint: arthro_____

7. resembling the sternum: stern_____

8. dissolution of a verterbra: spondylo_____

9. formation of bone marrow: myelo_____

10. cartilage softening: chondro_____

## Finding the Word Parts

Break each of the following terms into words or word parts. Give the definition of the term as well as the meaning of each word or word part.

1. rhadbdomyosarcoma: _____

_____

2. chondrodysplasia: _____

_____

3. pelviscope: _____

_____

4. osteoarthritis: _____

_____

5. cephalomegaly: _____

_____

6. patellectomy: _____

_____

7. fibromyalgia: _____

_____

8. cervicothoracic: _____

_____

9. ischioneuralgia: _____

_____

10. spondylosyndesis: _____

_____

## Proofreading and Understanding Terms

Write the correct spelling and definition in the blank to the right of any misspelled words. If the spelling is correct, write C.

1. oteoporossis: _____

2. mandible: _____

3. ossikle: _____

4. femor: _____

5. cartilage: _____

6. fibbia: _____

7. synovial: _____

8. cominuted fracture: _____

9. multiple scelrosis: _____

10. bursitis: _____

11. metatarsul: _____

12. falanges: _____

13. artroscopy: _____

14. ganglian: _____

15. fascia: _____

The following patient chart is used as a basis for a referral letter. Proofread the referral letter on page 56. There are five mistakes. Give corrections for the five errors in the space below and mark a category for each one. [A = minor spelling error; B = error that will cause someone else to have to check the information for accuracy; C = error that is potentially harmful to the patient.

1. _____

2. _____

3. _____

4. _____

5. _____

Patient: Deborah Pace          Date: 3/21/07          Time: 3:30

BP 120/60
T 98
Pulse 78

*Chief complaint: psoriasis; moles*

*Examined moles on leg. Top mole appears suspicious. Psoriasis spreading since last visit—referral to dermatologist for*

*further evaluation.*

*Amanda Liu, MD*

---

Dear Dr. Adams:

Dr. Liu has referred Deborah Pine to you for evaluation. She was last seen in our office on January 5, 2007 and has two complaints.

1. Two moles on her leg that are not suspicious.
2. Psoriasis on her arms that is recurrent.

Also, please note that her temperature was high although I found no sign of infection. Please let me know the results of your examination.

Sincerely,

Amanda Liu, MD

## Fill in the Blanks

1. A repetitive motion condition is called _____ syndrome.

2. The release of fluid or gas from the thorax is done by _____.

3. Skeletal muscles are _____ muscles.

4. Cardiac muscle is _____ muscle.

5. ROM stands for _____.

6. Surgical removal of a limb or part of a limb is _____.

7. The procedure of _____ is used to pull bone into alignment.

8. The part of a muscle attached to bone is the _____.

9. The collapse of a vertebra onto itself is called a _____ fracture.

10. In early childhood, most fractures are _____ fractures.

11. A check for bone density is used in the diagnosis of _____.

12. Tapping on a tendon as on the knee causes an automatic _____.

13. An agent that relieves muscle spasm is called a(n) _____.

14. An alternative medicine practitioner who works on manipulation and alignment of bone is a(n) _____.

15. A foot doctor is a(n) _____.

16. Abnormally slow muscle movement is _____.

17. A fluid-filled sac near a synovial joint is a(n) _____.

18. High levels of uric acid may indicate _____.

19. An osteoma is a tumor of _____.

20. A thin bone in the lower leg is the _____.

## True or False

Circle T for true or F for false.

1. The fontanels fuse before birth.     T     F

2. The palatine bones are in the middle ear.     T     F

3. An atrophied muscle moves easily.     T     F

4. Multiple sclerosis is not necessarily an inherited disease.     T     F

5. Rheumatoid arthritis appears only in adults.     T     F

6. Overexertion of a muscle may cause a strain.     T     F

7. Scoliosis affects the bones of the legs.     T     F

8. The skull has many sinuses.     T     F

9. The meniscus is a pad of cartilage.     T     F

10. The calcaneus is the largest bone in the hand.     T     F

## Write the Medical Term

For each of the following descriptions, write the proper medical term.

1. hunchback: _____

2. foot doctor: _____

3. broken bone: _____

4. kneecap: _____

5. wrist: _____

6. ankle: _____

7. thigh bone: _____

8. lower jaw: _____

9. upper jaw: _____

10. breastbone: _____

11. elbow: _____

12. swayback: _____

13. fingers or toes: _____

14. shin bone: _____

15. heel: _____

## Word Find

In the following puzzle, draw a line around at least 20 words pertaining to the integumentary system. The words can be horizontal, vertical, diagonal, or upside-down. Write the words on the rules provided. If you do not know the meaning of a word, look it up in your allied health dictionary and make a flash card for future review.

| | | | | | | | | | | | | | | | | | | |
|---|---|---|---|---|---|---|---|---|---|---|---|---|---|---|---|---|---|---|
| z | h | r | h | a | b | d | o | m | y | o | m | a | t | l | a | s | b | b | y |
| y | t | x | u | h | k | i | e | g | l | o | p | n | c | r | q | e | r | b | v |
| j | k | o | s | l | i | t | h | a | b | w | t | u | l | n | a | c | u | m | e |
| c | a | r | t | i | l | a | g | e | t | m | g | v | m | n | y | n | l | r | y |
| v | b | i | e | l | n | z | b | y | e | a | h | d | j | k | i | v | t | e | k |
| f | n | g | x | r | w | u | j | k | m | l | t | e | d | o | i | o | p | h | t |
| l | p | i | i | c | d | b | s | k | e | l | i | y | n | b | d | j | t | y | e |
| m | x | n | a | o | t | a | h | t | j | e | d | q | x | n | r | q | h | p | r |
| e | o | g | e | n | b | r | w | b | r | o | t | h | i | s | i | s | o | o | b |
| r | n | g | c | d | t | t | e | t | r | u | e | r | i | b | s | t | r | t | y |
| u | t | i | e | y | v | h | f | s | i | s | v | c | s | u | y | k | a | o | v |
| t | y | a | a | l | n | r | r | h | u | g | t | s | e | r | c | n | x | n | a |
| c | v | c | n | e | t | i | n | o | k | a | e | x | v | s | b | o | u | i | m |
| a | d | p | k | l | u | t | r | c | p | n | a | f | j | e | c | i | y | a | k |
| r | a | e | e | f | c | i | t | a | l | l | c | k | s | c | a | t | o | c | b |
| f | w | l | n | o | x | s | h | k | y | n | a | t | e | t | j | a | i | e | k |
| e | q | v | i | s | c | o | q | t | b | d | s | s | u | o | h | c | u | t | t |
| t | r | i | r | s | i | z | v | o | y | r | t | o | t | m | e | i | d | a | s |
| r | o | s | s | a | r | t | c | w | e | z | i | a | j | y | b | f | u | b | l |
| l | j | o | t | v | e | s | o | m | o | n | n | r | g | r | a | i | z | u | k |
| p | e | l | e | c | t | r | o | m | y | o | g | r | a | m | a | s | i | l | t |
| m | e | g | h | n | c | v | s | y | e | i | o | t | f | h | e | s | q | u | x |
| o | t | g | h | n | c | y | i | l | p | t | o | p | x | a | r | o | b | m | h |
| c | a | l | c | i | u | m | e | p | a | t | e | l | l | a | y | k | x | a | b |
| n | t | g | k | l | n | m | z | a | w | t | y | r | n | n | i | a | r | p | s |
| i | h | i | l | b | o | n | e | g | r | a | f | t | i | n | g | y | b | m | e |
| t | y | n | m | o | p | d | x | a | r | y | n | f | u | i | j | k | c | t | m |
| s | c | t | j | i | b | o | n | e | h | e | a | d | n | i | m | a | t | i | v |

List all the words you find in the word find on page 59 next to a letter a. through z. If you find more than 26 words, continue the list with aa. through zz on a separate sheet of paper. You will use these words in the next exercise.

a. _____

b. _____

c. _____

d. _____

e. _____

f. _____

g. _____

h. _____

i. _____

j. _____

k. _____

l. _____

m. _____

n. _____

o. _____

p. _____

q. _____

r. _____

s. _____

t. _____

u. _____

v. _____

w. _____

x. _____

y. _____

z. _____

## Match the Body Parts

For each of the following body parts, put at least two words from your Word Find results in the previous exercise. You could put a medical name, the abbreviation of where it is located, a diagnostic test related to that body part, or a disease.

skull: _____  _____

shoulder: _____  _____

wrist: _____  _____

arm: _____  _____

foot: _____  _____

leg: _____  _____

hip: _____  _____

thorax: _____  _____

nose: _____  _____

ear: _____ _____

mouth: _____ _____

## Crossword (Clues are on page 62.)

## CLUES

### Across

1. Shoulder bone

3. Bone pain

5. Inflammation of the joints

8. Long thigh bone

10. Parella

11. Slight, bony elevation

13. Device to measure angle of motion

15. Part of the scapula

17. Type of fracture

19. Involuntary movement

22. Bone _____

24. Physician who gives manipulative treatment

25. Lower leg bone

27. Portion of the hip bone

29. _____ fluid

31. Joining of two bone parts

34. Ring of bone at the base of the trunk

36. Muscle tumor

37. Joint repair

### Down

1. Collar bone

2. _____ disk

3. Incision into bone

4. Depression in the hip bone

6. Back portion of the foot

7. Bony structure

9. Stiffening

12. Vitamin D deficiency

14. Imaging of a joint

16. Intentional breaking of a bone

18. Bone formed in a tendon

20. Artificial device

21. Section of long bone

23. First crevical vertebra

26. Joining place of two bones

28. Removal of a bursa

30. Bony segments of the spine

32. _____ acid test

33. Combining form meaning spine

35. Nasal septum bone

A student at Essex Middle School, Jessica Chen, was injured in a soccer game.  The injury was not an emergency so the student rested in the nurse's office while waiting to be picked up by a parent. The school nurse wrote the following notes on a chart. From the notes, determine the body part that was damaged and describe the injury.

---

Essex Middle School
Nurse: <u>Joan Wiley</u>

Date: _____

Incident: <u>Jessica Chen was brought in by Amy Ellison with an ulnar bruise following a</u> <u>collision with another student on the soccer field. The site is swollen and Jessica is in</u> <u>severe pain. She is being transported to the emergency room for an x-ray.</u>

---

Body part injured: _____

_____

_____

_____

# A Practitioner's Day

The exercises that follow will take you through the few weeks following Jessica's injury.

## Contacting the Doctor

Jessica's mother called Dr. Wiley, Jessica's pediatrician. Laurie, the office receptionist, listened to the problem and went to Dr. Wiley to report the injury. Dr. Wiley decided to take the call as he was just between patients. He recommended that ice packs be used for the evening and that Jessica be given an over-the-counter NSAID as needed. He then instructed Laurie to schedule an appointment for the morning. Laurie fit Jessica in at 10:00 the next morning.

## The Visit

Laurie pulls Jessica's chart as she is setting up the day. At 10:00, Jessica has her appointment with Dr. Wiley. After the examination, he talks to Jessica and her father about how to handle the injury and what to expect. Jessica is a trained gymnast and usually spends two hours every day practicing for upcoming competitions. She will need to take at least a week off from intensive practice but Dr. Wiley thinks that she should go to the Sports Medicine center to see a massage therapist to get some relief and help her get back to her routine as soon as possible.

## The Massage Therapist

Steven Ruiz is the massage therapist who treats many of the gymnasts in town. Jessica's father calls for an appointment. Steven works in a sports medicine complex. Aside from two medical doctors, there are offices for a physical therapy practice and an x-ray facility. Steven's office is a small two-room suite. He is a sole practitioner but shares some part-time office help with the physical therapist. Many of his referrals come from local doctors and he makes sure to write a thank-you letter each time a new client is referred.

Since Jessica is a new client and Dr. Wiley has sent him a number of new clients, Steven takes care to show his gratitude in a letter he sends off after Jessica's first appointment.

On Steven's letterhead below, write an appropriate thank-you letter.

**Steven Ruiz**
Licensed Massage Therapist
688 Redwood Drive
Santa Ana, CA 88888
777-888-9999

Dear Dr. Wiley:

_____

_____

_____

_____

_____

_____

_____

_____

_____

_____

_____

_____

Sincerely,

Steven Ruiz

Since Jessica was just recently injured, Steven will use a very gentle Swedish massage for the first visit just to relax the injured area and relieve some of the pain. He schedules Jessica for a series of 8 appointments over the next 4 weeks to help her ease back into her routine. Jessica's parents' have medical insurance but it does not cover massage therapy. They agree to pay at each visit.

Steven has a steady stream of clients for 4 hours after Jessica's appointment. He won't have time to catch up on paperwork until he has a break from 3:00 to 3:45. During that time, he opens his mail, enters notes into the computer, answers phone messages, and gets some clerical work together for the clerk in the physical therapist's office.

Steven finds 3 messages from people needing to schedule or cancel appointments. He has found that the best way to handle it is to make a call slip for each message and have them in front of him as he returns the calls. Below are the 3 call slips. Write down a brief paragraph to describe the introduction to each returned call Steven will make.

Name: Allen Rodney

Phone: 667-7788

Message: needs to cancel appointment and reschedule

Name: Marisa Williams

Phone: 455-5555

Message: new patient, referred by Dr. Wiley, wants to find out about your services.

Name: Dr. Wiley

Phone: 333-4545

Message: Would like to discuss a patient with MS to see what you can do for spasticity.

Jessica's mother has given Steven a check for $30.00 for the first visit. He wrote her a hand receipt and has a copy for his files. Steven has 7 checks to deposit. He will make a deposit on the way home from the office. Here are the check amounts. Fill in the deposit slip for the bank.

   $ 60.35

   $ 42.00

   $ 30.00

   $ 75.00

   $106.00

   $ 22.00

Midway Bank

Account No. 54567809098

Date: _____

| | |
|---|---|
| Cash | |
| Checks (list separately) | |
| | |
| | |
| | |
| | |
| | |
| Total | |

# Terms in the Cardiovascular System

## Word Parts in the Cardiovascular System

These are the major word parts used to form words in the cardiovascular system. When you combine these parts with some of the prefixes and suffixes in Units 2 and 3, you will be able to understand medical terms relating to the cardiovascular system.

| | |
|---|---|
| angi(o) | blood vessel |
| aort(o) | aorta |
| arteri(o), arter(o) | artery |
| ather(o) | fatty matter |
| atri(o) | atrium |
| cardi(o) | heart |
| hemangi(o) | blood vessel |
| pericardi(o) | pericardium |
| phleb(o) | vein |
| sphygm(o) | pulse |
| thromb(o) | blood clot |
| vas(o) | blood vessel |
| ven(o) | vein |

After practicing word building and terminology exercises related to the cardiovascular system, you will meet a patient with symptoms of a heart attack as he calls his physician and goes to the hospital for treatment.

## Exercises in the Cardiovascular System

### Building Terms

For each of the following definitions, provide a term using cardiovascular system word parts as well as prefixes and suffixes you learned in Units 2 and 3.

1. pertaining to both the atrium and ventricles: _____

2. development of new blood vessels: _____

3. hardening of the arteries: _____

4. disease of the vascular and nervous systems: _____

5. pertaining to arteries and veins: _____

6. breaking up of a thrombus: _____

7. softening of the heart muscle: _____

8. heart inflammation: _____

9. benign tumor filled with blood vessels: _____

10. hardening of the walls of a vein: _____

11. relaxation of a blood vessel: _____

12. of the heart and lungs: _____

13. blood vessel suture: _____

14. vein inflammation with the presence of a blood clot: _____

15. surgical repair of a blood vessel: _____

16. diagnostic testing that records electrical heart impulses: _____

17. puncture of the pericardium: _____

18. valve repair: _____

19. faulty heart rhythm: _____

20. enlarged heart: _____

## Completing Terms

Complete the following terms by adding a prefix or suffix to the word or word part given here.

1. arising from the heart: cardio _____

2. creation of a surgical opening in the pericardium: percardio _____

3. x-ray image of a vein: phlebo _____

4. disease of the heart muscle: cardiomyo _____

5. between two ventricles: _____ ventricular

6. membrane that covers the myocardium: _____ cardium

7. smooth inner layer of blood vessels: _____ thelium

8. agent that lowers blood pressure: _____ hypertensive

9. inflammation within an artery: _____ carditis

10. agent that breaks up clots: _____ coagulant

## Finding the Word Parts

Break each of the following terms into words or word parts. Give the definition of the term as well as the meaning of each word or word part.

1. cardiorrhexis: _____

_____

2. thromboplebitis: _____

_____

3. myocardium: _____

_____

4. atherosclerosis: _____

_____

5. echocardiogram: _____

_____

6. endarterectomy: _____

_____

7. electrocardiogram: _____

_____

8. angiocardiography: _____

_____

9. atrioventricular: _____

_____

10. phlebotomy: _____

_____

## Proofreading and Understanding Terms

Write the correct spelling and definition in the blank to the right of any misspelled words. If the spelling is correct, write C.

1. auscultation: _____

2. embalus: _____

3. diastolyc: _____

4. systolic: _____

5. protrombin: _____

6. infarction: _____

7. ventrikle: _____

8. pericardiom: _____

9. capillery: _____

10. aneurysm: _____

The following insurance card is being used to input an electronic bill to a company for collection. The data that is input also follows. Proofread the data and find any errors.

HealthCare Solutions
www.hcsol.com

Name(s)

Granger, Stewart D.   01
Granger, Alicia M.     02
Granger, Sarah M.      03
Granger, Peter B.      04

Elec. Claim Payer ID#
8877799

Company
**Pace Electric, Inc.**

Subscriber / Group
6788890909 / 5TYS145

Data

_____

_____

_____

_____

Patient: Stuart D. Grainger

Insurance: United Care Solutions

Employer: Pace Financial

Subscriber # 6878890909

## Fill In the Blanks

1. The largest artery in the body is the _____.

2. A small vein is a(n) _____.

3. Blood pressure is measured with a(n) _____.

4. The _____ node helps to set the heart rate.

5. The _____ artery carries blood to the leg.

6. Circulation between the heart and lungs is _____ circulation.

7. The fetal heart has an opening in the septum called the _____ _____.

8. The largest veins in the body are the superior and inferior _____ _____.

9. Heart pain is _____.

10. An area of dead tissue is _____.

11. Four congenital heart defects are known as the _____ of Fallot.

12. A backflow of blood into a valve is known as _____.

13. Absence of a heartbeat is _____.

14. Cardiac _____ are measured during a myocardial infarction.

15. Cholesterol levels are checked in a _____ profile.

16. Cardiac _____ is a diagnostic procedure to evaluate heart function.

17. The _____ valve is between the right atrium and the right ventricle.

18. The wall dividing the heart is the _____.

19. The layer of heart muscle is the _____.

20. The rhythmic heart contractions can be felt as the _____.

## True or False

Circle T for true or F for false.

1. A venule is an enlarged vein.     T     F

2. Bradycardia is an excessively slow rhythm.     T     F

3. Arteriosclerosis indicates the artery's normal state.     T     F

4. A CBC is the most common blood test.     T     F

5. Blood flows through arteries toward the heart.     T     F

6. Blood flows through veins away from the heart.     T     F

7. The mitral valve is also called the biscuspid valve.     T     F

8. The endocardium is the sac enclosing the heart.     T     F

9. The popliteal artery is in the leg.     T     F

10. The lumen is a build-up of fatty material in an artery.     T     F

11. In vasoconstriction, the smooth muscle tightens.     T     F

12. An axillary pulse is felt in the neck.     T     F

13. The heart's rhythm is coordinated in the conduction system.     T     F

14. A blood clot is often treatable with medication.     T     F

15. Tachycardia is an abnormally slow heart rate.     T     F

16. LDL is considered "good" cholesterol.     T     F

17. A stress test measures psychological stress on the heart.     T     F

18. X-ray image of a blood vessel is an angiogram.     T     F

19. A stent is usually placed in veins.     T     F

20. Aneurysms are usually caused by a build-up of plaque.     T     F

## Write the Medical Term

For each of the following descriptions, write the proper medical term.

1. heart attack: _____

2. high blood pressure: _____

3. low blood pressure: _____

4. rapid heart rate: _____

5. slow heart rate: _____

6. blood clot in a vein or an artery: _____

7. fatty deposit in an artery: ___ _____

## Crossword (Clues are on page 74.)

## CLUES

### Across

1. Artery inflammation

3. Carry oxygenated blood

4. Fatty substance

7. One unit of pulse

9. _____ inhibitor

11. Combining form for muscle

13. _____ maker

14. Tiny blood vessel

15. Partition between heart chambers

17. _____

18. Heart sound heard on auscultation

19. Localized blood insufficiency

23. Largest artery

24. _____ arteriosus

25. Device that regulates the heart beat

26. _____ cardiogram

28. Frictional sound heard on auscultation

29. Upper right heart chamber

31. High = _____ lipoprotein

32. Chest pain

33. High blood pressure

### Down

1. Largest artery

2. Contraction phase of blood pressure

3. Of the atrium

5. Channel inside artery

6. Goal of lower cholesterol

8. Abnormally fast heart rate

10. Bluish coloration

12. Place where blood enters the heart from systemic circulation

16. Muscular layer of heart tissue

18. Bicuspid valve

20. Muscular organ that circulates blood

21. Abnormally slow heart rate

22. Abbreviation for atrial fibrillation

27. Implanted tissue

28. Pace of heart beat

30. _____ blood pressure

## Find the Meaning

In the following article about health, pick out the terms that refer to the cardiovascular system and define each one.

---

What are the health consequences of overweight for children and teens?

Children and teens who are overweight may begin to experience health consequences during their youth as well as putting themselves at risk for weight-related health problems later in life.

Overweight children and teens have been found to have risk factors for cardiovascular disease, including high cholesterol, elevated insulin levels, and elevated blood pressure during childhood. One study showed that approximately 60% of overweight children had a least one cardiovascular risk factor, such as high cholesterol or high blood pressure; in comparison, only 10% of children with healthy weight had at least one risk factor. Additionally, 25% of overweight children had two or more risk factors.

Other health consequences include the following potential problems:

- Type 2 diabetes
- Potential for early arteriosclerosis
- Sleep apnea (not breathing for at least 10 seconds during sleep)
- Social consequences including poor self-esteem and social discrimination

_____

_____

_____

_____

_____

_____

---

## Dealing with an Emergency

The exercises that follow will take you through a patient case study for this unit. The patient is *Giovanni Elio.* He is 55 years old and has taken the day off from work because he has what he describes as a bad case of indigestion. Giovanni feels worse as the day progresses. He calls his physician and describes the indigestion as well as a tingling in his arm. His doctor tells him to get to the emergency room immediately. Giovanni's wife drives him to the hospital, which is six blocks away.

## Fill in the Blanks

At the emergency room, Giovanni was taken in right away for evaluation while his wife filled out paperwork at the reception area. She filled in all the patient information and was asked for a(n) _____ card. She was asked to read and sign a document detailing the privacy policy of the hospital. In addition to name, address, and phone number, she was asked to provide her husband's _____ number.

After filling in all the forms, Mrs. Elio went into the treatment area where she was told that her husband was being stabilized after having a heart attack. She was told he was being moved to the cardiac care unit on the third floor.

## Cardiac Care Unit

After Giovanni was admitted to the cardiac care unit, his wife was allowed to see him for a brief time. Mrs. Elio was issued a visitor's pass at the information center in the reception area of the hospital. On it was her name and the floor she was visiting. Upon reaching the third floor, Mrs. Elio went to the nurse's desk. There, she introduced herself to the nurse on duty who directed her to room 322.

## Introducing Yourself

The nurse on duty, Jane Callahan, greets Mrs. Elio and asks you (the nursing assistant) to escort Mrs. Elio to room 322. You introduce yourself. Write down how you would introduce yourself to her.

_____

_____

_____

_____

After you reach the room, you ask her if there is anything else you can do right now. She says "not at the moment." She thanks you, and you leave.

## The Daily Routine

As a nursing assistant, you keep notes of your interactions with patients every day making every effort to complete the log as you go. By the end of your shift, you have added a lot of notes. The log is used by all the nursing assistants on all shifts so you must remember to be neat and accurate.

You performed the following tasks. Add them to the log in the appropriate place.

1. While Mr. Elio was taken downstairs for a procedure at 10:30, you changed his bed.

2. At the same time, you changed his catheter bag and emptied 30 cc of urine.

3. Mr. Elio is on a special diet. His prepared tray was delivered to the floor and you served it at 12:15.

4. You collected his tray at 12:40 and noticed that he had only eaten his applesauce—and nothing else. You notified the nurse and put it in the log.

5. You gave Mr. Elio a bed bath at 2:00.

| March 29, 2008/Time | Patient | Provider | Services Performed |
|---|---|---|---|
| 8:00-8:30 | | | |
| 8:30-9:00 | | | |
| 9:00-9:30 | | | |
| 9:30-10:00 | | | |
| 10:00-10:30 | | | |
| 10:30-11:00 | | | |
| 11:00-11:30 | | | |
| 11:30-12:00 | | | |
| 12:00-12:30 | | | |
| 12:30-1:00 | | | |
| 1:00-1:30 | | | |
| 1:30-2:00 | | | |
| 2:00-2:30 | | | |
| 2:30-3:00 | | | |
| 3:00-3:30 | | | |
| 3:30-4:00 | | | |
| 4:00-4:30 | | | |
| 4:30-5:00 | | | |

## Communicating with the Patient

You have been taught to talk to the patient and explain everything you are going to do. Write a brief conversation about what you might say to Mr. Elio before and during the bed bath.

_____

_____

_____

_____

_____

## Looking for a Job

Your hospital hours are only part-time and you have heard that a home health care agency is hiring CNAs for weekend work. Compose a resume similar to the one shown in Unit 1 on page 10.

_____
_____
_____

OBJECTIVE: _____

SUMMARY: _____
_____
_____
_____
_____

EDUCATION: _____
_____

EXPERIENCE: _____
_____
_____
_____
_____
_____
_____
_____

ACTIVITIES: _____
_____

## Interview

You get a call from Sunshine and schedule an interview for Thursday morning before you go to work at the hospital. After being introduced to the manager, you are asked about your skills and what job you seek. Write a brief paragraph giving an introductory statement to the manager.

_____

_____

_____

_____

# Terms in the Respiratory System

## Word Parts in the Respiratory System

These are the major word parts used to form words in the respiratory system. When you combine these parts with some of the prefixes and suffixes in Units 2 and 3, you will be able to understand medical terms relating to the respiratory system.

| | |
|---|---|
| adenoid(o) | adenoid, gland |
| alveol(o) | alveolus |
| bronch(o), bronchi(o) | bronchus |
| bronchiol(o) | bronchiole |
| capn(o) | carbon dioxide |
| epiglott(o) | epiglottis |
| laryng(o) | larynx |
| lob(o) | lobe of the lung |
| mediastin(o) | mediastinum |
| nas(o) | nose |
| or(o) | mouth |
| ox(o), oxi-, oxy- | oxygen |
| pharyng(o) | pharynx |
| phon(o) | voice, sound |
| phren(o) | diaphragm |
| pleur(o) | pleura |
| pneum(o), pneumon(o) | air, lung |
| rhin(o) | nose |
| spir(o) | breathing |
| steth(o) | chest |
| thorac(o) | thorax, chest |
| tonsill(o) | tonsils |
| trache(o) | trachea |

After practicing word building and terminology exercises related to the respiratory system, you will follow a respiratory therapist through a day on the job.

## Exercises in the Respiratory System

### Building Terms

For each of the following definitions, provide a term using respiratory system word parts as well as prefixes and suffixes you learned in Units 2 and 3.

1. pertaining to the bronchi and lungs: _____

2. air in the chest cavity: _____

3. inflammation of the larynx, trachea, and bronchi: _____

4. excessive rate of respiration: _____

5. surgical puncture of the chest cavity: _____

6. creation of an opening in the trachea: _____

7. incision into the trachea: _____

8. nose inflammation: _____

9. ear, nose, and throat specialist: _____

10. insufficient oxygen: _____

11. puncture of the pleural cavity: _____

12. removal of a nerve controlling the diaphragm: _____

13. narrowing of a bronchus: _____

14. blood in the chest cavity: _____

15. softening of the bronchi: _____

16. involving the chest and the abdomen: _____

17. tracheal inflammation with pus: _____

18. of the nose and tear glands: _____

19. inflammation of the epiglottis: _____

20. widening of the bronchi: _____

## Completing Terms

Complete the following terms by adding a prefix or suffix to the word or word part given here.

1. normal or good breathing: _____ pnea

2. difficult breathing: _____ pnea

3. sudden contraction of the bronchi: broncho _____

4. abnormally slow breathing: _____ pnea

5. abnormally fast breathing: _____ pnea

6. between the ribs: _____ costal

7. lung specialist: pulmono _____

8. bronchial dilation: bronchi _____

9. bluish skin condition: cyan _____

10. within the trachea: _____ tracheal

11. cough suppressant: _____ tussive

12. opening in the trachea: tracheo _____

13. removal of the tonsils: tonsil _____

14. excess carbon dioxide in the blood: _____ capnia

15. difficulty speaking: _____ phonia

16. tool to examine the larynx: laryngo _____

17. without oxygen: _____ oxia

18. relating to an alveolus: alveoli _____

19. any chronic lung disease: pneumoni _____

20. pain in the chest: pleuro _____

## Finding the Word Parts

Break each of the following terms into words or word parts. Give the definition of the term as well as the meaning of each word or word part.

1. hypoxemia: _____

_____

**2.** bronchodilator: _____

_____

**3.** tracheobronchial: _____

_____

**4.** pleurocentesis: _____

_____

**5.** pyothorax: _____

_____

**6.** pneumococcus: _____

_____

**7.** hemoptysis: _____

_____

**8.** anoxia: _____

_____

**9.** spirometer: _____

_____

**10.** orthopnea: _____

_____

**11.** pneumolith: _____

_____

**12.** pleurodesis: _____

_____

**13.** bronchoconstriction: _____

_____

**14.** tracheorrhagia: _____

_____

15. oromandibular: _____

_____

16. phrenalgia _____

_____

17. bronchioloalveolar: _____

_____

18. oxyhemoglobin: _____

_____

19. broncholithiasis: _____

_____

20. stethoscope: _____

_____

## Proofreading and Understanding Terms

Write the correct spelling and definition in the blank to the right of any misspelled words. If the spelling is correct, write C.

1. atilectstasis: _____

2. emphysema: _____

3. Hiemlich maneuver: _____

4. phyranx: _____

5. tachypnia: _____

6. penumonia: _____

7. anthrakosis: _____

8. expectorent: _____

9. laryngal: _____

10. inspiration: _____

Proofread the cover letter you are sending for a job. Find any typing or spelling errors and list and correct them here.

---

Dear Ms. Stanton:

This letter is in response to the advertesment you placed on the website careerbuilder. com. As you can see from the attached risume, my experience as a respiretiory therapist is right in line with what you are seeking. I would appreciate hearing from you and look forward to meeting you to discuss the positon.

Thank you for your consideration.

Sincerly yours,

Andrew Ethan

---

_____

_____

_____

_____

_____

_____

## Fill In the Blanks

1. Carbon dioxide and air are exchanged in the part of the lungs called the _____.

2. Exhalation and breathing in is also called _____.

3. The _____ contracts and expands during breathing.

4. During exhalation, a gas, _____ _____, is expelled.

5. The _____ is the passageway between the larynx and the bronchi.

6. Another name for the throat is the _____.

7. The left lung has two _____.

8. The _____ is the top part of each lung.

9. A risk factor for lung cancer is _____.

10. Inflammation of the lung membranes is _____.

## True or False

Circle T for true or F for false.

1. An agent that promotes productive coughing is an expectorant.    T    F

2. Bronchitis is a chronic lung infection.    T    F

3. Rales are high-pitched squeaking sounds.    T    F

4. Cystic fibrosis is contagious.    T    F

5. Asbestosis is caused by working with coal.    T    F

6. An oximeter measures respiration.    T    F

7. CPR ventilates the lungs.    T    F

8. Auscultation is a common blood test.    T    F

9. Asthma is sometimes treated with corticosteriods.    T    F

10. SARS is a hereditary disease.    T    F

## Write the Medical Term

For each of the following descriptions, write the proper medical term.

1. black lung disease: _____

2. sore throat: _____

3. runny nose: _____

4. chest cold: _____

5. spitting up of blood: _____

6. spit: _____

7. whooping cough: _____

8. cough suppressant: _____

9. breathing in: _____

10. breathing out: _____

# Crossword

## CLUES

### Across

1. External breathing structure

3. Membrane on the outside of the lungs

5. _____ sample

7. Hiccuping

9. Their vibrations produce sound

12. Bronchial narrowing condition

14. Popping sounds

17. Combining form for lung

18. Windpipe

21. Organ of voice production

23. Oxygen deficiency

24. Acute alveolar infection

25. Whistling sounds on inspiration

27. Abnormally deep breathing

30. Combining form for mouth

33. Combining form for breath

35. Middle section of the right lung

36. A nasal divider

### Down

1. Inflammation of the nose and pharynx

2. Paranasal cavity

3. Of the lung

4. Air sacs in the lungs

5. Lung condition

6. Rare type of lung cancer

8. High-pitched respiratory sound

10. Hairlike extensions

11. Division of the pharynx

13. Procedure to prevent choking

15. Organ of respiration

16. Abnormally slow breathing

19. Inflammation of the pleura

20. To breathe out

22. Exhalation

25. Trachea

26. Lymphoid tissue in the nasopharynx

27. Midsection of the lung

28. Of the thorax

29. One section of the lung

31. Pharynx

32. Peak _____

34. Crackles

## Research a Disease

Either using the Internet or using reference books in the library, write a paragraph on asthma, including what it is, how it is controlled, and potential new developments in the control and cure of this disease.

_____

_____

_____

_____

_____

_____

_____

# A Day on the Job

The exercises that follow will take you a day as a respiratory therapist working for a home care agency. You will do all the patient interaction, reporting, and colleague interaction that takes place in a typical day.

## Keeping a Log

The home care agency you work for schedules clients throughout the day. You have to log in all visits, mileage, work done and time spent. On Monday, you see 6 clients and perform the following tasks. The distances and times are listed here.

**8:30 Mary Vasquez:** 8 miles from your home. Mary receives oxygen therapy. You change her tank, check her equipment, and interview her about her therapy to see if she is comfortable.

**9:45 John Autemont:** 10.6 miles from Mary's home. John lives in a senior citizen's complex. He has just recovered from pneumonia and has chronic bronchitis. He receives oxygen therapy at home. You check his tank which will not need changing and you talk to him about his bronchitis. Because he seems to be having trouble today, you give him some of his inhaler through a special machine as directed by his physician who has said he should be given this therapy twice a day as needed. Because he is struggling, you will return at 4:00 to give him another treatment.

**11:00 Peter Walters:** Lives in the same complex as John. He uses a ventilator which needs cleaning and inspection twice a month. Today is one of those visits. You will also interview Peter about how he is doing.

**12:30-1:15:** Lunch break

**1:30 Billy Williams:** Lives 7 miles from the complex and has cystic fibrosis. You visit every couple of weeks to work with the family who has to help him cough up mucus to clear his lungs. Today, you watch his mother do the procedure and help when it appears that Billy is struggling.

**2:15 Jeanette Dixon:** 4 miles from Billy, an 80-year-old woman who lives with her daughter and has emphysema. You check her oxygen and interview her.

**3:30 Ella Simmons:** Lives in the same senior complex (11 miles from the Dixon home) where John Autemont lives, has congestive heart failure, is bedridden because of a viral infection, and gets oxygen therapy. You check her equipment and interview her.

**4:00 John Autemont:** A return for another inhaler treatment and to see how he is doing. This was not scheduled but you called in to the agency to confirm that you should add this visit to your schedule.

| Monday | Patient | Provider | Services Performed |
|---|---|---|---|
| 8:00-8:30 | | | |
| 8:30-9:00 | | | |
| 9:00-9:30 | | | |
| 9:30-10:00 | | | |
| 10:00-10:30 | | | |
| 10:30-11:00 | | | |
| 11:00-11:30 | | | |
| 11:30-12:00 | | | |
| 12:00-12:30 | | | |
| 12:30-1:00 | | | |
| 1:00-1:30 | | | |
| 1:30-2:00 | | | |
| 2:00-2:30 | | | |
| 2:30-3:00 | | | |
| 3:00-3:30 | | | |
| 3:30-4:00 | | | |
| 4:00-4:30 | | | |
| 4:30-5:00 | | | |

## Using the Phone

During the day, you must make a number of telephone calls. There is no need for you to call homebound clients who expect your visit. However, in the case of Billy Williams, you call 15 minutes before you go there to confirm the appointment. Write a short paragraph giving the call you might make to Billy's mother.

_____

_____

_____

_____

Your supervisor at the agency is Paul Bronstein. Call him in the morning after you see John Autemont and ask him for permission to return at 4:00. Write your end of the conversation below.

_____

_____

_____

_____

## Getting Reimbursed

At the end of each week, you submit your hours and mileage for payment. Using the billing form below, write down your Monday hours and miles.

| Day | Hours | Miles | Provider | Supervisor's Signature |
|-----------|-------|-------|----------|------------------------|
| Monday    |       |       |          |                        |
| Tuesday   |       |       |          |                        |
| Wednesday |       |       |          |                        |
| Thursday  |       |       |          |                        |
| Friday    |       |       |          |                        |
| Saturday  |       |       |          |                        |
| Sunday    |       |       |          |                        |
| TOTALS    |       |       |          |                        |

# Terms in the Nervous System

## Word Parts in the Nervous System

These are the major word parts used to form words in the nervous system. When you combine these parts with some of the prefixes and suffixes in Units 2 and 3, you will be able to understand medical terms relating to the nervous system.

| | |
|---|---|
| cerebell(o) | cerebellum |
| cerebr(o), cerebri- | cerebrum |
| crani(o) | cranium |
| encephal(o) | brain |
| -esthesia | sensation, feeling |
| gangli(o) | ganglion |
| gli(o) | neuroglia |
| mening(o), meningi(o) | meninges |
| myel(o) | bone marrow, spinal cord |
| neur(o), neuri- | nerve |
| -paresis | weakness |
| -plegia | paralysis |
| psycho- | mind |
| radiculo- | nerve root |
| spin(o) | spine |
| thalam(o) | thalamus |
| vag(o) | vagus nerve |
| ventricul(o) | ventricle |

After practicing word building and terminology exercises related to the nervous system, you will learn about working with a client with multiple sclerosis who lives at home.

# Exercises in the Nervous System

## Building Terms

For each of the following definitions, provide a term using nervous system word parts as well as prefixes and suffixes you learned in Units 2 and 3.

1. pertaining to nerves and muscles: _____

2. chemical messenger that sends nerve impulses: _____

3. paralysis on one side: _____

4. hardening of the brain: _____

5. complete paralysis: _____

6. of a blood vessel in the brain: _____

7. disorder with sudden episodes of falling asleep: _____

8. condition with tumors arising from nerve tissue: _____

9. instrument for measuring the skull: _____

10. brain inflammation: _____

11. surgical cutting of a nerve root: _____

12. any disease affecting both the brain and spinal cord: _____

13. inflammation of the brain and meninges: _____

14. relating to the spine and nerves: _____

15. disease of the nerve roots: _____

## Completing Terms

Complete the following terms by adding a prefix or suffix to the word or word part given here.

1. paralysis of all four limbs: _____plegia

2. weakness on only one side: _____paresis

3. softening of the bones of the skull: cranio_____

4. difficulty with reading and writing: _____lexia

5. surgical opening in a ventricle: ventriculo_____

6. brain inflammation: encephal_____

7. within a ventricle: _____ventricular

8. abnormally heightened sensation: _____esthesia

9. inflammation of many nerves: _____neuritis

10. nerve disease: neuro_____

11. agent for prevent of seizures: _____epileptic

12. incision into the skull: cranio_____

13. inflammation of a nerve root: radicul_____

14. surgical cutting of the vagus nerve: vago_____

15. tumor of the meninges: meningi_____

16. without a brain: _____encephaly

17. cutting of nerve fibers: cordo_____

18. loss of ability to speak: _____phasia

19. one-half of the brain: _____sphere

20. mentally confused: _____oriented

## Finding the Word Parts

Break each of the following terms into words or word parts. Give the definition of the term as well as the meaning of each word or word part.

1. paraesthesia: _____

_____

2. myelomalacia: _____

_____

3. electroencephalogram: _____

_____

4. meningomyelitis: _____

_____

5. neurosurgery: _____

_____

6. myelofibrosis: _____

_____

Name _____

Class _____ Date _____

7. psychomotor: _____

_____

8. myelomeningocele: _____

_____

9. cerebrospinal: _____

_____

10. craniocele: _____

_____

11. meningorrhagia: _____

_____

12. cranioschisis: _____

_____

13. encephalomyeloradiculitis: _____

_____

14. meningococcus: _____

_____

15. myelodysplasia: _____

_____

## Proofreading and Understanding Terms

Write the correct spelling and definition in the blank to the right of any misspelled words. If the spelling is correct, write C.

1. neuralgia: _____

2. gliobalastoma: _____

3. meninges: _____

4. cerbral palsy: _____

5. Alzhimers disease: _____

6. dora mater: _____

7. tregiminal: _____

8. myelogram: _____

9. encephalitis: _____

10. anasthesia: _____

11. acetilcholene: _____

12. myelin: _____

13. axen: _____

14. dandrite: _____

15. neuroglia: _____

## Find the Error

A patient with multiple sclerosis (MS) is being released from the hospital after a major flare-up. In the hospital, she was treated with corticosteroids and is now being given discharge instructions that include the exact instructions for tapering down. Below is a portion of her chart and of the discharge instructions. Describe any inconsistencies you find between the two.

Patient: <u>Mary Pelton</u>                                    Date: October 10, 2009

Attending Physician: <u>Robert Walker</u>

<u>Flare-up reduced—patient to be released today. Continue antibiotics for 7 days. See</u>
<u>neurologist for follow-up within 1 week. Important for patient to stay cool—no hot</u>
<u>showers, avoid sun for lengthy periods. Over-the-counter pain killers should be limited</u>
<u>to no more than 4 per day.</u>

_____

_____

_____

_____

October 10, 2009

Discharge instructions for: <u>Mary Pelton</u>

ACTIVITIES:

    1. You may resume normal outdoor activity as soon as you are able.

    2. If you feel weak or dizzy, rest and call your neurologist.

MEDICATIONS

    1. Continue the antibiotic in your discharge package for 4 days.

    2. Take Tylenol as needed.

FOLLOW-UP

Schedule an appointment with your neurologist within the next two weeks.

_____

_____

_____

_____

_____

_____

## Filling in the Blanks

1. The three layers of the meninges are the _____ mater, the arachnoid, and the _____ mater.

2. Efferent nerves carry impulses _____ from the spinal cord.

3. An individual nerve cell is a(n) _____.

4. The _____ nervous system commands involuntary bodily functions.

5. The body's own natural pain relievers are neurotransmitters called _____.

6. Total loss of memory is _____.

7. Lack of oxygen during birth may cause _____ palsy.

8. Paralysis on one side is _____.

9. A(n) _____ is an unconscious state caused by trauma.

10. Another word for a seizure is a(n) _____.

## True or False

Circle T for true or F for false.

**1.** The trigeminal nerve moves the lower extremities.     T     F

**2.** The central nervous system consists of the brain and spinal cord.     T     F

**3.** Alzheimer's disease is caused by a bacteria.     T     F

**4.** An epidural is a type of anesthesia.     T     F

**5.** A reflex is a voluntary muscle reaction.     T     F

**6.** Brain wave patterns can be seen on an EKG.     T     F

**7.** A lumbar puncture is also called a spinal tap.     T     F

**8.** Babinski's sign is a test for sciatic nerve damage.     T     F

**9.** Craniotomy is the removal of a spinal disk.     T     F

**10.** Serotonin is only a chemically manufactured agent.     T     F

## Using a Dictionary

Using your allied health dictionary, go to the combining form *cranio-*. Find five words that use that word root. Break them down into word parts and give the definition of each word.

**1.** _____

_____

**2.** _____

_____

**3.** _____

_____

**4.** _____

_____

**5.** _____

_____

## Writing the Medical Term

For each of the following descriptions, write the proper medical term.

1. water on the brain: _____

2. stroke: _____

3. someone who is totally crippled: _____

4. neuralgia: _____

5. total forgetfulness: _____

6. split personality: _____

7. headache: _____

8. sudden attack: _____

9. violent head blow: _____

10. severe leg pain: _____

## Word Find

In the following puzzle, draw a line around at least 20 words pertaining to the integumentary system. The words can be horizontal, vertical, diagonal, or upside-down. Write the words on the rules provided. If you do not know the meaning of a word, look it up in your allied health dictionary and make a flash card for future review.

```
y  s  p  e  l  i  p  e  y  j  k  o  k  e  c  g  n  i  t  o
l  c  e  p  a  r  e  s  t  h  e  s  i  a  p  r  a  x  i  a
s  e  v  e  n  h  u  s  t  n  f  k  p  a  x  c  i  t  s  v
z  r  e  h  u  m  k  u  a  m  b  a  g  n  o  s  i  a  p  s
s  e  z  b  n  j  m  k  y  q  e  r  x  m  y  u  s  v  i  o
e  b  n  k  m  f  y  e  m  u  i  n  a  r  c  f  w  a  n  m
v  r  j  c  l  a  l  a  n  w  r  g  y  u  j  i  i  v  r  n
r  a  d  b  g  i  s  n  j  i  y  a  u  l  a  s  c  a  a  a
e  l  s  o  t  n  d  i  v  e  n  e  u  r  o  s  v  g  v  m
n  c  g  i  q  t  w  i  n  e  b  g  o  v  a  u  e  o  j  b
l  o  s  t  m  i  t  q  s  b  l  e  i  v  n  r  n  t  z  u
a  r  x  v  a  n  n  t  j  y  k  i  b  t  q  e  t  o  e  l
n  t  i  a  g  g  h  r  n  m  q  w  c  z  i  y  r  m  k  i
i  e  o  n  m  e  e  t  h  a  l  a  m  u  s  s  i  y  q  s
p  x  x  z  t  b  s  a  w  y  n  c  o  r  d  v  c  n  j  m
s  n  e  i  s  u  l  o  b  o  t  o  m  y  a  c  l  t  b  y
j  a  c  z  c  j  t  y  c  k  s  n  w  u  i  d  e  n  m  e
m  a  n  l  u  o  n  e  r  v  e  c  e  l  l  a  c  o  y  m
c  n  u  g  n  o  s  s  z  n  u  u  j  d  r  y  e  i  a  b
i  s  s  n  e  u  r  o  n  s  a  s  s  y  b  e  a  t  y  o
t  i  c  h  r  l  y  x  d  o  c  s  l  n  e  q  f  u  s  l
o  t  m  y  s  l  a  p  p  y  t  i  c  k  t  v  i  l  c  u
c  i  g  a  p  v  e  q  c  i  t  o  n  p  y  h  v  o  e  s
r  r  h  n  o  o  d  z  t  e  b  n  h  y  p  n  o  v  o  x
a  u  h  u  n  d  w  v  u  j  g  q  x  n  m  k  s  n  z  h
n  d  n  e  s  p  i  n  a  l  c  o  r  d  i  t  i  o  c  h
y  u  c  x  a  e  v  y  k  k  n  b  t  u  j  c  e  c  k  a
y  m  l  i  p  y  h  p  a  r  g  o  n  m  o  s  y  l  o  p
```

a. _____    e. _____

b. _____    f. _____

c. _____    g. _____

d. _____    h. _____

i. _____        r. _____

j. _____        s. _____

k. _____        t. _____

l. _____        u. _____

m. _____        v. _____

n. _____        w. _____

o. _____        x. _____

p. _____        y. _____

q. _____        z. _____

# A Day in the Life of a CNA

## Helping a Client at Home

Leila Ramsey is 40 years old and has multiple sclerosis. She was diagnosed in her early 20s and managed fairly well until age 38 with only a gradual decline. At first, she limped a little, then she used a cane but was able to get to work easily, drive, go out, and maintain her life independently. In the past two years, however, the disease has progressed rapidly to the point where Leila needs an aide daily for about two hours in the morning and two hours at night. Because Leila is still working, the state provides the aide along with van services that transport her to work and doctor's appointments. You are a certified nursing assistant employed by the state and Leila is your responsibility for four hours every day, Monday through Friday. On the weekends, another aide takes over.

## Dealing with the Client as an Individual

You report into the state department of rehabilitative services by telephone daily and more if needed. You also go there in person every Thursday at 2:00 for a meeting with your supervisor. As a certified nursing assistant, you have been trained in certain tasks. You must also be a skilled communicator—able to deal with clients, keep careful records for the state, and able to report clearly and accurately to your supervisor.

You are on your way to Leila's home for the first time. Your supervisor will meet you there along with Leila's mother who has been helping Leila for the past month while the state has made arrangements for Leila's home care.

Your supervisor, Elisa Velasquez, introduces you to Leila and her mother. Together, all four of you discuss Leila's routine and what services you will provide. You are given a key to the home so you can enter and you take Leila's cell phone number and home number and give her both of your phone numbers.

## At-Home Care Tasks

Using the Internet or the library, look up the skills that a CNA might need to use for a client in Leila's situation. Describe at least five tasks in the space below.

_____

_____

_____

_____

_____

_____

_____

## Communication with Your Client

Communication with a client is important. Leila is sometimes discouraged and angry. On the third day when you arrive, Leila is very angry and takes it out on you. How would you respond if Leila tells you to just shut up?

_____

_____

_____

_____

Once you and Leila have worked out this difficult time, the work continues but you have been told to report such incidents to your supervisor. Write a brief paragraph describing the above incident to your supervisor.

_____

_____

_____

_____

Leila goes to an acupuncturist who has been helping her with pain management. She asks you to make an appointment at a time when you can take her. Describe the call you will make to Dr. Chen's office.

_____

_____

_____

_____

## Keeping Your Log Current

Fill out your weekly log just for the work you did with Leila.

Client: _____ Provider: _____ Week of: _____

| Monday | Tuesday | Wednesday | Thurday | Friday |
|--------|---------|-----------|---------|--------|
| 8:00-8:30 | 8:00-8:30 | 8:00-8:30 | 8:00-8:30 | 8:00-8:30 |
| 8:30-9:00 | 8:30-9:00 | 8:30-9:00 | 8:30-9:00 | 8:30-9:00 |
| 9:00-9:30 | 9:00-9:30 | 9:00-9:30 | 9:00-9:30 | 9:00-9:30 |
| 9:30-10:00 | 9:30-10:00 | 9:30-10:00 | 9:30-10:00 | 9:30-10:00 |
| 10:00-10:30 | 10:00-10:30 | 10:00-10:30 | 10:00-10:30 | 10:00-10:30 |
| 10:30-11:00 | 10:30-11:00 | 10:30-11:00 | 10:30-11:00 | 10:30-11:00 |
| 11:00-11:30 | 11:00-11:30 | 11:00-11:30 | 11:00-11:30 | 11:00-11:30 |
| 11:30-12:00 | 11:30-12:00 | 11:30-12:00 | 11:30-12:00 | 11:30-12:00 |
| 12:00-12:30 | 12:00-12:30 | 12:00-12:30 | 12:00-12:30 | 12:00-12:30 |
| 12:30-1:00 | 12:30-1:00 | 12:30-1:00 | 12:30-1:00 | 12:30-1:00 |
| 1:00-1:30 | 1:00-1:30 | 1:00-1:30 | 1:00-1:30 | 1:00-1:30 |
| 1:30-2:00 | 1:30-2:00 | 1:30-2:00 | 1:30-2:00 | 1:30-2:00 |
| 2:00-2:30 | 2:00-2:30 | 2:00-2:30 | 2:00-2:30 | 2:00-2:30 |
| 2:30-3:00 | 2:30-3:00 | 2:30-3:00 | 2:30-3:00 | 2:30-3:00 |
| 3:00-3:30 | 3:00-3:30 | 3:00-3:30 | 3:00-3:30 | 3:00-3:30 |
| 3:30-4:00 | 3:30-4:00 | 3:30-4:00 | 3:30-4:00 | 3:30-4:00 |
| 4:00-4:30 | 4:00-4:30 | 4:00-4:30 | 4:00-4:30 | 4:00-4:30 |
| 4:30-5:00 | 4:30-5:00 | 4:30-5:00 | 4:30-5:00 | 4:30-5:00 |

# UNIT 9

# Terms in the Urinary System

## Word Parts in the Urinary System

These are the major word parts used to form words in the urinary system. When you combine these parts with some of the prefixes and suffixes in Units 2 and 3, you will be able to understand medical terms relating to the urinary system.

| | |
|---|---|
| cyst(o) | bladder, especially the urinary bladder |
| meat(o) | meatus |
| nephr(o) | kidney |
| pyel(o) | renal pelvis |
| ren(o) | kidney |
| ur(o), urin(o) | urine |
| ureter(o) | ureter |
| urethr(o) | urethra |
| -uria | of urine |
| vesic(o) | bladder, generally used when describing something in relation to a bladder |

After practicing word building and terminology exercises related to the urinary system, you will learn about working for a specialist who deals with problems of the urinary system.

## Exercises in the Urinary System

### Building Terms

For each of the following definitions, provide a term using urinary system word parts as well as prefixes and suffixes you learned in Units 2 and 3.

1. blood in the urine: _____

2. cancerous tumor of the kidney: _____

3. condition with build-up of pus in a ureter: _____

4. painful urination: _____

5. albumin in the urine: _____

6. falling down of the kidney from its proper position: _____

7. dilation of the ureter: _____

8. hardening of the kidneys: _____

9. blood in the urine: _____

10. removal of a kidney stone: _____

11. of the bladder and vagina: _____

12. inflammation of both the urethra and the urinary bladder: _____

13. malignant kidney tumor: _____

14. instrument to examine a meatus: _____

15. x-ray of the renal system: _____

## Completing Terms

Complete the following terms by adding a prefix or suffix to the word or word part given here.

1. of the space behind the peritoneum: _____ peritoneal

2. kidney-shaped: nephr _____

3. abnormal narrowing of a ureter: uretero _____

4. hernia in the bladder: vesico _____

5. glucose in the urine: glycos _____

6. absence of urine: _____ uria

7. plastic surgery of the urethra: urethra _____

8. surgical fixing of the kidney: nephro _____

9. bladder suture: cysto _____

10. calculus in the urinary tract: cysto _____

11. surgical attachment of the ureters to an opening in the intestines: ureteroileo _____

12. Kidney condition: nephr _____

13. incision to enlarge a meatus: meato _____

14. surgical removal of a kidney stone through the renal pelvis: pyelolitho _____

15. painful urination: uro _____

## Finding the Word Parts

Break each of the following terms into words or word parts. Give the definition of the term as well as the meaning of each word or word part.

1. genitourinary: _____

_____

2. nephrolithiasis: _____

_____

3. glomerulonephritis: _____

_____

4. ureteritis: _____

_____

5. cystourethrography: _____

_____

6. lithotripsy: _____

_____

7. nephroptosis: _____

_____

8. hemodialysis: _____

_____

9. proteinuria: _____

_____

10. cystadenoma: _____

_____

11. ureteropyelonephritis: _____

_____

12. nephrosonography: _____

_____

13. pyeloureteritis: _____

_____

14. urolithiasis: _____

_____

15. vesicocele: _____

_____

## Proofreading and Understanding Terms

Write the correct spelling and definition in the blank to the right of any misspelled words. If the spelling is correct, write C.

1. erythopoietin: _____

2. hypospadius: _____

3. enuresis: _____

4. nephrectomy: _____

5. diouretic: _____

6. nefron: _____

7. glomerulus: _____

8. incontenance: _____

9. lithotrypsy: _____

10. urethritis: _____

11. trigon: _____

12. uremia: _____

13. policystic: _____

14. ascites: _____

15. cystitis: _____

## Reading for Details

The urinalysis shown below indicates several abnormal readings. Go over the lab results carefully and list those things that are abnormal.

Name _____

Class _____ Date _____

---

Dr. Joel Chorzik
1420 Glen Road
Meadowvale, OK 44444
111-222-3333

Run Date: 09/22/XX
Run Time: 1507

Page 1
Specimen Report

| Patient: James Delgado | Acct #: A994584732 | Loc: ED | U #: |
| Reg Dr: S. Anders, M.D. | Age/Sx: 55/M | Room: | Reg: 09/22/XX |
| | Status: Reg ER | Bed: | Des: |

| Spec #: 0922 : U0009A | Coll: 09/22/XX | Status: Comp | Req #: 77744444 |
| | Recd.: 09/22/XX | Subm Dr: | |

Entered: 09/22/XX–0841          Other Dr:
Ordered: UA with micro
Comments: Urine Description: Clean catch urine

| Test | Result | Flag | Reference |
|------|--------|------|-----------|
| *Urinalysis* | | | |
| *UA with micro* | | | |
| COLOR | YELLOW | | |
| APPEARANCE | HAZY | ** | |
| SP GRAVITY | 1.018 | | 1.001-1.030 |
| GLUCOSE | NORMAL | | NORMAL mg/dl |
| BILIRUBIN | NEGATIVE | | NEG |
| KETONE | NEGATIVE | | NEG mg/dl |
| BLOOD | 2+ | ** | NEG |
| PH | 5.0 | | 4.5-8.0 |
| PROTEIN | TRACE | ** | NEG mg/dl |
| UROBILINOGEN | NORMAL | | NORMAL-1.0 mg/dl |
| NITRITES | NEGATIVE | | NEG |
| LEUKOCYTES | 2+ | ** | NEG |
| WBC | 20-50 | ** | 0-5 /HPF |
| RBC | 2-5 | | 0-5 /HPF |
| EPI CELLS | 20-50 | | /HPF |
| BACTERIA | 2+ | ** | |
| MUCUS | | | |

Patient 1

_____

_____

_____

_____

_____

_____

## Filling in the Blanks

1. The kidneys are located in the _____ space.

2. A(n) _____ is used to drain urine.

3. The kidneys are surrounded by the _____.

4. The inside of the bladder contains folds called _____.

5. A cystourethrogram is an image of the bladder and the _____.

6. A permanent catheter is used in _____ dialysis.

7. A Foley catheter is a type of _____ catheter.

8. A procedure to break up stones is extracorporeal shock wave _____.

9. Overactive bladder is treated with a(n) _____ agent.

10. A specialist who treats kidney disorders is a(n) _____

11. A scanty urine production is _____.

12. A malignant kidney tumor that occurs in children is _____.

13. Cloudy or turbid urine indicates a(n) _____.

14. The urine of people with uncontrolled diabetes will contain _____.

15. A specialist who treats urinary tract disorders is a(n) _____.

## True or False

Circle T for true or F for false.

1. Pyuria is excessive urination.     T     F

2. It is possible to live with only one kidney.     T     F

3. The hilum is another name for the renal artery.     T     F

4. The trigone is an area of the bladder.     T     F

5. The loop of Henle is part of the kidney.     T     F

6. The kidneys remove waste material from the blood.     T     F

7. Urea goes from the kidneys into the blood stream.     T     F

8. Cystitis occurs most frequently in men.     T     F

9. Epispadias is a birth defect with the meatus located on the underside of the penis.     T     F

10. Nocturia is excessive daytime urination.     T     F

11. Urine is cultured to detect infections.     T     F

12. A BUN is a test that monitors kidney function.     T     F

13. Drug screening is usually done in a CBC.     T     F

14. Before a kidney transplant, it is necessary to have a nephrectomy.     T     F

15. A kidney stone may cause renal colic.     T     F

## Using a Dictionary

Your allied health dictionary is a primary tool for learning the correct pronunciation. If your dictionary has an audio CD with pronunciations, look up the following five terms in the dictionary, pronounce them from the pronunciation given, and then check your pronunciations by listening to the audio CD. If your dictionary does not have an audio CD, ask your instructor to listen to your pronunciations.

1. urinalysis

2. catheter

3. nephrologist

4. urethrostomy

5. micturition

## Writing the Medical Term

For each of the following descriptions, write the proper medical term.

1. passing water (give 3 possibilities): _____, _____,

   _____

2. kidney stone: _____

3. bladder stone: _____

4. painful urination: _____

5. blood in the urine: _____

Name _____

Class _____ Date _____

## Word Find

In the following puzzle, draw a line around at least 20 words pertaining to the integumentary system. The words can be horizontal, vertical, diagonal, or upside-down. Write the words on the rules provided. If you do not know the meaning of a word, look it up in your allied health dictionary and make a flash card for future review.

| k | i | d | n | e | y | r | e | d | d | a | l | b | y | r | a | n | i | r | u |
|---|---|---|---|---|---|---|---|---|---|---|---|---|---|---|---|---|---|---|---|
| h | a | b | r | t | d | a | n | s | b | r | e | n | i | n | t | y | a | r | j |
| x | b | l | o | f | a | s | t | j | u | n | v | a | b | i | t | i | t | s | w |
| j | k | i | c | s | t | s | h | j | k | l | m | t | r | s | r | j | l | e | x |
| a | n | t | i | p | a | s | m | o | d | i | c | t | a | r | i | b | t | d | z |
| e | r | h | n | c | y | x | a | t | u | k | l | l | n | y | g | u | o | e | s |
| u | r | o | c | k | a | n | s | d | w | e | p | i | c | n | o | s | u | m | e |
| r | x | t | i | h | m | g | y | c | c | o | w | u | a | j | n | x | e | a | i |
| e | n | o | t | y | e | k | l | r | l | q | t | e | r | h | e | p | z | c | m |
| t | q | m | e | g | h | j | k | e | k | l | h | d | l | e | c | o | p | e | e |
| e | h | y | r | o | c | o | y | a | c | o | r | t | e | x | t | f | y | k | n |
| r | a | q | u | b | j | p | i | t | l | c | o | p | a | e | k | h | u | n | u |
| a | x | e | i | b | v | r | j | i | k | l | s | y | m | n | z | w | r | t | r |
| n | h | e | d | m | z | e | t | n | u | k | k | i | u | i | u | r | e | a | e |
| e | a | z | w | i | n | m | o | e | p | s | a | i | t | g | h | j | k | i | s |
| p | a | m | e | a | t | u | s | l | o | i | b | n | b | i | s | r | y | d | i |
| h | l | i | t | y | s | c | v | n | r | m | u | r | e | h | r | k | l | p | s |
| r | e | n | o | g | r | a | m | u | g | v | a | m | u | l | i | h | y | j | k |
| o | x | c | r | g | h | y | t | j | l | x | h | v | b | h | d | t | p | w | k |
| m | n | b | m | e | t | a | t | s | o | r | p | x | e | e | t | f | b | e | r |
| a | a | e | v | m | m | h | d | u | r | i | c | n | m | n | i | a | s | x | n |
| m | j | i | v | e | d | c | i | e | t | j | e | k | l | o | x | i | p | n | k |
| a | z | s | h | x | r | j | c | k | n | q | e | s | x | t | m | r | u | e | o |
| c | y | s | t | o | p | l | a | s | t | y | d | x | o | e | e | u | x | p | i |
| s | f | t | y | w | n | u | c | i | v | a | c | t | k | c | m | g | b | h | w |
| q | n | o | c | t | u | r | i | a | u | r | e | m | i | a | u | i | u | r | j |
| c | b | y | u | i | s | a | r | c | c | m | h | y | r | x | a | l | r | o | k |
| z | y | g | o | l | o | r | u | r | i | n | e | w | i | o | p | o | g | n | x |

a. _____    e. _____

b. _____    f. _____

c. _____    g. _____

d. _____    h. _____

i. _____    r. _____

j. _____    s. _____

k. _____    t. _____

l. _____    u. _____

m. _____    v. _____

n. _____    w. _____

o. _____    x. _____

p. _____    y. _____

q. _____    z. _____

# Working in a Specialist's Office

Jim Balboa is a billing clerk in the Urology Associates office located in the medical center attached to the local hospital. There are three urologists in the busy practice. Jim is the only billing clerk but there is an office manager, a receptionist, and a medical assistant. All four of the office people work together to make sure the office runs smoothly. The receptionist is the first in line to answer the phone but rollover calls go to Jim next and then to the other two workers. That way, unless there is an unusual volume of calls, all calls are answered within three rings. Jim also sits at the reception desk for an hour each day while the receptionist is at lunch.

On Tuesday, the three urologists see 36 patients. Jim has a lot of bills to enter. He uses an electronic billing system. He receives the superbills from the medical assistant and he enters the information into the billing system. He also keeps track of payments as they come in and pursues the collection of payments due.

## Entering Superbill Data

On the next two pages are a superbill and a screen for a patient who has been seen previously. Fill in the correct information into the computer.

*Allen Medical Center*
*14 Center St.*
*Stokesville, NY 00006*
*777-888-9999*

☐ PRIVATE ☐ BLUECROSS ☐ IND. ☐ MEDICARE ☐ MEDICAID ☐ HMO ☐ PPO

| PATIENT'S LAST NAME | FIRST | ACCOUNT # | BIRTHDATE | SEX ☑ MALE | TODAY'S DATE |
|---|---|---|---|---|---|
| Fortuna | Leonard | 79623 | 08/14/73 | ☐ FEMALE | 01/31/09 |

| INSURANCE COMPANY | SUBSCRIBER | PLAN # | SUB. # | GROUP # |
|---|---|---|---|---|
| Wellcare, Ltd. | Safenet, Inc. | | XY284 | 86082 |

ASSIGNMENT: I hereby assign my insurance benefits to be paid directly to the undersigned physician. I am financially responsible for non-covered services.
SIGNED: (Patient)
Parent (if Minor) Len Fortuna          DATE:    01 / 31 / 09

RELEASE: I hereby authorize the physician to release to my insurance carriers any information requested to process this claim.
SIGNED: (Patient)
Parent (if Minor) Sen Fortune          DATE:    01 / 31 / 09

| ✓ | DESCRIPTION | CPT/Med | Dx/Re | PEE | ✓ | DESCRIPTION | CPT/Med | Dx/Re | PEE | ✓ | DESCRIPTION | CPT/Med | Dx/Re | PEE |
|---|---|---|---|---|---|---|---|---|---|---|---|---|---|---|
| | OFFICE CARE | | | | | PROCEDURES | | | | | INJECTIONS/IMMUNIZATIONS | | | |
| | NEW PATIENT | | | | | Treadmill (in Office) | 93015 | | | | Tetanus | | 90718 | |
| | Brief | 99201 | | | | 24-hour Holter | 93224 | | | | Hypertet | J1870 | 90782 | |
| | Limited | 99202 | | | | if Medicare set-up fee | 93225 | | | | Pneumococcal | | 90732 | |
| | Intermediate | 99203 | | | | Physician Interpret | 93227 | | | | Influenza | | 90724 | |
| | Extended | 99204 | | | | EKG w/Interpretation | 93000 | | | | TB Skin Test (PPD) | | 86585 | |
| | Comprehensive | 99205 | | | | EKG (Medicare) | 93005 | | | | Antigen Injection-Single | | 95115 | |
| | | | | | | Sigmoidoscopy | 45300 | | | | Multiple | | 95117 | |
| | ESTABLISHED PATIENT | | | | | Sigmoidoscopy (flexible) | 45330 | | | | B12 Injection | J3420 | 90782 | |
| | Minimal | 99211 | | | | Sigmoidos., Flex. w/Bx. | 45331 | | | | Injection, IM | | 90782 | |
| | Brief | 99212 | | | | Spirometry FEV/FVC | 94010 | | | | Compazine | J0780 | 90782 | |
| | Limited | 99213 | | | | Spirometry, Post-Dilator | 94080 | | | | Demerol | J2175 | 90782 | |
| | Intermediate | 99214 | | | | | | | | | Vistaril | J3410 | 90782 | |
| | Extended | 99215 | | | | | | | | | Susphrine | J0170 | 90782 | |
| | Comprehensive | 00215 | | | | LABORATORY | | | | | Decadron | J0890 | 90782 | |
| | | | | | ✓ | Blood Draw Fee | 36415 | | | | Estradiol | J1000 | 90782 | |
| | CONSULTATION-OFFICE | | | | | Urinalysis, chemical | 81005 | | | | Testosterone | J1080 | 90782 | |
| | Focused | 99241 | | | | Throat Culture | 87081 | | | | Lidocaine | J2000 | 90782 | |
| | Expanded | 99242 | | | | Occult Blood | 82270 | | | | Solumedrol | J2920 | 90782 | |
| | Detailed | 99243 | | | | Pap Handling Charge | 99000 | | | | Solucortel | J1720 | 90782 | |
| | Comprehensive 1 | 99244 | | | | Pap Life Guard | 88150-90 | | | | Hydeltra | J1680 | 90782 | |
| | Comprehensive 2 | 99245 | | | | Gram Stain | 87205 | | | | Pen procaine | H2510 | 90788 | |
| | | | | | | Hanging Drop | 87210 | | | | INJECTIONS-JOINT/BURSA | | | |
| | | | | | | Urine Drug Screen | 99000 | | | | Small Joints | | 20800 | |
| | | | | | | | | | | | Intermediate | | 20605 | |
| | | | | | | SUPPLIES | | | | | Large Joints | | 20810 | |
| | | | | | | | | | | | Trigger Point | | 20550 | |
| | | | | | | | | | | | MISCELLANEOUS | | | |

| DIAGNOSIS: | ICD-9 | | | | | | | | |
|---|---|---|---|---|---|---|---|---|---|
| __ Abdominal Pain | 789.0 | ✓ Gout | 274.0 | __ C.V.A. -Acute | 436. | __ Electrolyte Dis. | 276.9 | __ Herpes Simplex | 054.9 |
| __ Abscess (Site) | 682.9 | __ Asthma | 493.90 | __ Cere. Vas. Accid. (Old) | 438 | __ Fatigue | 780.7 | __ Herpes Zoster | 053.9 |
| __ Adverse Drug Rx | 995.2 | __ Asthmatic Bronchitis | 493.90 | __ Cerumen | 380.4 | __ Fibrocys. Br. Dis. | 610.1 | __ Hydrocele | 603.9 |
| __ Alcohol Detox | 291.8 | __ Atrial Fib | 427.31 | __ Chestwall Pain | 786.59 | __ Fracture (Site) | 829.0 | __ Hyperlipidemia | 272.4 |
| __ Alcoholism | 303.90 | __ Atrial Tachi | 427.0 | __ Cholecystitis | 575.0 | __ Open/Close | | __ Hypertension | 401.9 |
| __ Allergic Rhinitis | 477 | __ Bowel Obstruct. | 560.9 | __ Cholelithiasis | 574.00 | __ Fungal Infect. (Site) | 110.8 | __ Hyperthyroidism | 242.9 |
| __ Allergy | 995.3 | __ Breast Mass | 611.72 | __ COPD | 492.8 | __ Gastric Ulcer | 531.90 | __ Hypothyroidism | 244.9 |
| __ Alzheimer's Dis. | 290.1 | __ Bronchitis | 490 | __ Cirrhosis | 571.5 | __ Gastritis | 535.0 | __ Labyrinthitis | 386.30 |
| __ Anemia | 285.9 | __ Bursitis | 727.3 | __ Cong. Heart Fail. | 428.9 | __ Gastroenteritis | 558.9 | __ Lipoma (Site) | 214.9 |
| __ Anemia-Pernicious | 281.0 | __ Cancer, Breast (Site) | 174.9 | __ Conjunctivitis | 372.30 | __ G.I. Bleeding | 578.9 | __ Lymphoma | 202.8 |
| __ Angina | 413.9 | __ Metastatic (Site) | 199.1 | __ Contusion (Site) | 924.9 | __ Glomerulonephritis | 583.9 | __ Mit. Valve Prolapse | 424.0 |
| __ Anxiety Synd. | 300.00 | __ Colon | 153.9 | __ Costochondritis | 733.99 | __ Headache | 784.0 | __ Myocard. Infarction (Area) | 410.9 |
| __ Appendicitis | 541 | __ Cancer, Rectal | 154.1 | __ Depression | 311. | __ Headache, Tension | 307.81 | __ M.I., Old | 412 |
| __ Arteriosl. H.D. | 414.0 | __ Lung (Site) | 162.9 | __ Dermatitis | 692.9 | __ Migrane (Type) | 346.9 | __ Myositis | 729.1 |
| __ Arthritis, Osteo. | 715.90 | __ Skin (Site) | 173.9 | __ Diabetes Mellitus | 250.00 | __ Hemorrhoids | 455.6 | __ Nausea/Vomiting | 767.0 |
| __ Rheumatoid | 714.0 | __ Card. Arrhythmia (Type) | 427.9 | __ Diabetic Ketosis | 250.1 | __ Hernia, Hiatal | 553.3 | __ Neuralgia | 729.2 |
| __ Lupus | 710.0 | __ Cardiomyopathy | 425.4 | __ Diverticulitis | 562.11 | __ Inguinal | 550.9 | __ Nevus (Site) | 216.9 |
| | | __ Cellulitis (Site) | 682.9 | __ Diverticulosis | 562.10 | __ Hepatitis | 573.3 | __ Obesity | 278.0 |

DIAGNOSIS: (IF NOT CHECKED ABOVE)

| SERVICES PERFORMED AT: | ☐ Office ☐ E.R. | ☐ CLAIM CONTAINS NO | REFERRING PHYSICIAN & I.D. NUMBER |
|---|---|---|---|
| ☐ | ☐ | ORDERED REFERRING SERVICE | |

| RETURN APPOINTMENT INFORMATION: | NEXT APPOINTMENT | ACCEPT | DOCTOR'S SIGNATURE |
|---|---|---|---|
| 5 - 10 - 15 - 20 - 30 - 40 - 60 | M - T - W - TH - F - S | ASSIGNMENT? | |
| | | AM  ☐ YES | |
| [    DAYS] [    WKS.] [    MOS.] [    PRN] DATE   /   /   TIME: | | PM  ☐ NO | |

| | |
|---|---|
| ☐ CASH | TOTAL TODAY'S FEE |
| ☐ CHECK # | OLD BALANCE |
| ☐ VISA | TOTAL DUE |
| ☐ MC | |
| ☐ CO-PAY | AMOUNT REC'D. TODAY |

1. Complete upper portion of this form, sign and date.
2. Attach this form to your own Insurance company's form for client reimbursement.

MEDICARE PATIENTS - DO NOT SEND THIS TO MEDICARE.
WE WILL SUBMIT THE CLAIM FOR YOU.

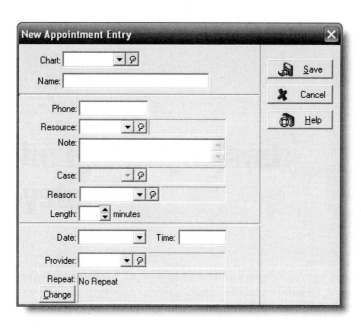

# UNIT 10

# Terms in the Female Reproductive System

## Word Parts in the Female Reproductive System

These are the major word parts used to form words in the female reproductive system. When you combine these parts with some of the prefixes and suffixes in Units 2 and 3, you will be able to understand medical terms relating to the female reproductive system.

| | |
|---|---|
| anmni(o) | amnion |
| cervic(o) | cervix |
| colp(o) | vagina |
| episi(o) | vulva |
| galact(o) | milk |
| gynec(o) | female |
| hyster(o) | uterus |
| lact(o), lacti- | milk |
| mamm(o), mamma- | breast |
| mast(o) | breast |
| men(o) | menstruation |
| metr(o) | uterus |
| oo | egg |
| oophor(o) | ovary |
| ov(o), ovi- | egg |
| ovari(o) | ovary |
| perine(o) | perineum |
| salping(o) | fallopian tube |
| uter(o) | uterus |
| vagin(o) | vagina |
| vulv(o) | vulva |

Name _____

Class _____ Date _____

After practicing word building and terminology exercises related to the female reproductive system, you will learn about working in a women's health center.

# Exercises in the Female Reproductive System

## Building Terms

For each of the following definitions, provide a term using female reproductive system word parts as well as prefixes and suffixes you learned in Units 2 and 3.

1. muscular lining of the uterus: _____

2. scanty menstrual flow: _____

3. pus in the fallopian tube: _____

4. following birth: _____

5. egg production: _____

6. around menopause: _____

7. surgical removal of the breast: _____

8. lack of ovulation: _____

9. abnormal discharge of breast milk: _____

10. inflammation of the vulva and vagina: _____.

11. first pregnancy: _____

12. removal of fluid from the amniotic sac: _____

13. removal of an ovary: _____

14. excessive menstrual flow: _____

15. woman who was never pregnant: _____

16. removal of the uterus: _____

17. breast pain: _____

18. immature egg cell: _____

19. surgical fixing of an ovary in position: _____

20. fungal infection of the vagina: _____

## Completing Terms

Complete the following terms by adding a prefix or suffix to the word or word part given here.

1. inner uterine lining: _____ metrium

2. visual examination of the vagina: colpo _____

3. before menstruation: _____ menstrual

4. newborn: _____ nate

5. before birth: _____ natal

6. inflammation of the fallopian tubes: salping _____

7. benign tumor of the myometrium: leiomy _____

8. lack of menstrual flow: _____ menorrhea

9. bending backward (as the uterus): _____ version

10. x-ray image of the breast: mammo _____

11. having borne many children: _____ parous

12. plastic surgery of the breasts: mamma _____

13. milk producing: lacti _____

14. specialty in treatment of newborns: neonato _____

15. uterine discharge: metro _____

16. painful menstruation: _____ menorrhea

17. leakage of amniotic fluid: amnio _____

18. end of menstruation: meno _____

19. uterine pain: metr _____

20. egg-shaped: ov _____

## Finding the Word Parts

Break each of the following terms into words or word parts. Give the definition of the term as well as the meaning of each word or word part.

**1.** mastoptosis: _____

_____

**2.** hysteratresia: _____

_____

**3.** galactopoiesis: _____

_____

**4.** metroperitonitis: _____

_____

**5.** oophorectomy: _____

_____

**6.** vaginolabial: _____

_____

**7.** uteropexy: _____

_____

**8.** episiotomy: _____

_____

**9.** colpoperineorrhaphy: _____

_____

**10.** hysterosalping-oophorectomy: _____

_____

## Proofreading and Understanding Terms

Write the correct spelling and definition in the blank to the right of any misspelled words. If the spelling is correct, write C.

1. ginecology: _____

2. estragen: _____

3. obstetrician: _____

4. perineum: _____

5. zygote: _____

6. volva: _____

7. preclampsia: _____

8. dysplasia: _____

9. embrio: _____

10. pediatrishun: _____

## Eliminating Confusion

The obstetrician you work for has asked you to set appointments for Molly T., who is three months pregnant at 42 years of age. Since it is her first pregnancy, she is at high risk. The doctor asks that you set up appointments for every three weeks for the months 4 through 6 and then every two weeks for months 7 and 8. The custom is to give the patient a card with the appointments listed on the back for three months in advance. Here is what you give her. What mistakes have you made?

Appointments for second trimester:

February 1 (beginning of month 4): 9:00

February 21: 10:15

March 21: 11:30

April 12: 9:00

April 26: 10:15

_____

_____

_____

## Filling in the Blanks

1. The domelike top of the uterus is the _____.

2. Beginning at nine weeks of gestation, the embryo is called the _____.

3. Nutrients in the womb are provided by the _____.

4. The _____ dilates during labor to allow passage of the head.

5. The first milk from the breasts is called the _____.

6. Uterine tissue in abnormal areas is called _____.

7. The falling down of the uterus from its normal position is called _____.

8. A common yeast infection of the vagina is _____.

9. A test for fetal abnormalities by withdrawing fluid from the sac is _____.

10. Fetuses are often viewed through _____.

## True or False

Circle T for true or F for false.

1. Most females are born with many millions of ovaries.     T     F

2. The beginning of menstruation is known as the menarche.     T     F

3. Progesterone is the major male hormone found also in females.     T     F

4. The fallopian tubes are where normal implantation takes place.     T     F

5. The endometrial lining is shed during menstruation.     T     F

6. Menopause usually starts at puberty.     T     F

7. Gestation is the period from conception to birth.     T     F

8. Meconium is the substance within the umbilical cord.     T     F

9. The area surrounding the breast nipple is the areola.     T     F

10. The dropping of the fetal head into position in the pelvis is called molding.     T     F

11. The climacteric is the stage prior to menopause.     T     F

12. Abruptio placentae is the sudden separation of the placenta from the uterine wall.     T     F

13. Milk engorgement in the breasts can cause mastitis.    T    F

14. Some forms of breast cancer have a hereditary component.    T    F

15. A Pap smear is a type of mammogram.    T    F

## Using a Dictionary

In your allied health dictionary, find five tests that examine the female reproductive system visually. (Hint: use the list of combining forms at the beginning of this unit to look for tests build with these word parts.) Give a short description of the purpose of each test.

1. _____

   _____

2. _____

   _____

3. _____

   _____

4. _____

   _____

5. _____

   _____

## Writing the Medical Term

For each of the following descriptions, write the proper medical term or an alternative medical term.

1. fallopian tube: _____

2. soft spot in the head: _____

3. womb: _____

4. spontaneous abortion: _____

5. period: _____

6. change of life: _____

7. cramps and discomfort before menstruation: _____

8. egg: _____

9. baby in the womb: _____

10. birth control: _____

## Word Find

In the following puzzle, draw a line around at least 20 words pertaining to the integumentary system. The words can be horizontal, vertical, diagonal, or upside-down. Write the words on the rules provided. If you do not know the meaning of a word, look it up in your allied health dictionary and make a flash card for future review.

| g | l | o | p | x | v | w | a | r | e | o | l | a | x | p | g | h | u | d | k |
|---|---|---|---|---|---|---|---|---|---|---|---|---|---|---|---|---|---|---|---|
| r | a | o | x | y | t | o | c | i | n | v | r | c | g | a | j | y | y | i | d |
| a | z | r | t | h | j | k | o | b | n | w | e | o | a | r | g | s | h | a | l |
| v | x | s | n | o | i | r | o | h | c | q | n | r | j | a | l | t | t | p | i |
| i | c | p | a | c | v | y | t | r | e | b | u | p | w | s | t | e | y | h | i |
| d | a | o | v | m | a | n | i | g | a | v | w | u | h | v | n | r | r | r | j |
| a | a | n | l | h | a | t | k | l | x | q | z | s | e | j | k | e | i | a | e |
| g | h | g | j | p | k | s | n | o | i | t | a | l | u | p | o | c | w | g | a |
| h | l | e | p | b | o | x | t | w | r | y | n | u | d | s | j | t | k | m | c |
| h | y | p | o | x | s | s | w | o | r | k | c | t | m | u | v | o | a | j | k |
| t | y | r | a | v | o | c | c | b | p | w | a | e | t | m | o | m | p | b | r |
| s | g | z | v | y | u | i | k | o | c | e | r | u | a | a | n | y | o | p | l |
| z | c | o | n | d | o | m | e | w | p | b | x | m | m | j | m | k | x | h | m |
| w | r | t | n | u | i | c | n | m | q | y | s | y | d | y | w | n | j | m | l |
| o | t | b | j | a | x | w | t | h | w | c | b | u | j | i | o | x | i | e | s |
| p | a | s | e | w | d | m | l | u | m | p | e | c | t | o | m | y | x | o | u |
| l | w | x | r | t | h | b | b | j | k | l | p | s | i | z | e | q | y | j | n |
| a | b | o | r | t | i | o | n | n | r | o | i | p | s | s | s | c | b | i | i |
| c | i | s | x | v | o | d | d | o | o | t | z | y | n | k | t | q | o | e | s |
| e | b | y | x | n | w | y | m | n | i | p | p | l | e | l | r | h | p | n | w |
| n | q | z | e | m | k | r | g | c | e | v | b | j | k | i | o | m | m | s | e |
| t | s | m | k | l | e | r | i | w | y | e | t | e | m | a | g | g | b | u | s |
| a | y | o | i | t | a | v | b | n | h | e | f | a | p | l | e | w | a | s | s |
| h | i | n | y | n | r | w | s | y | p | h | i | l | i | s | n | v | z | a | e |
| n | m | c | k | e | q | t | g | y | s | m | o | g | v | r | l | w | y | u | m |
| x | o | w | c | u | l | d | o | s | c | o | p | y | t | u | w | b | n | j | o |
| o | s | x | t | g | e | w | b | c | m | j | q | a | v | t | k | b | t | y | x |
| n | i | k | s | e | r | o | f | w | n | a | m | e | n | o | r | r | h | i | a |

a. _____        n. _____

b. _____        o. _____

c. _____        p. _____

d. _____        q. _____

e. _____        r. _____

f. _____        s. _____

g. _____        t. _____

h. _____        u. _____

i. _____        v. _____

j. _____        w. _____

k. _____        x. _____

l. _____        y. _____

m. _____        z. _____

## Working in a Women's Health Center

You are a mammography technician at the Greenville Women's Health Center. You generally have a full schedule of clients who will get a mammogram in the room where you work. Appointments are scheduled for 30 minutes to allow time for processing and for repeat imaging if necessary.

## Communicating with the Patient

For each appointment, the receptionist gives you the patient's folder. You go to the reception area and bring the patient to the mammography room. There you point out the gown she is to change in to and that you will be back in five minutes. Write a brief paragraph describing what you would say to Mary Altomonte when bringing her in to the room.

_____

_____

_____

_____

_____

_____

## Keeping Track

You then come back to the room and take 8 images which you process. Each time you take an image you check it and label it with the patient's name and date. After you are finished labeling, you fill out a form that accompanies the images to the radiologist. It is vital that there be no mix-ups.

Complete Mary Altomonte's form.

Name: _____ Lab Technician: _____

Date: _____ Number of Total Images: _____

# Terms in the Male Reproductive System

## Word Parts in the Male Reproductive System

These are the major word parts used to form words in the male reproductive system. When you combine these parts with some of the prefixes and suffixes in Units 2 and 3, you will be able to understand medical terms relating to the male reproductive system.

| | |
|---|---|
| andr(o) | men |
| balan(o) | glans penis |
| epididym(o) | epididymis |
| orch(o), orchi(o), orchid(o) | testes |
| prostat(o) | prostate gland |
| sperm(o), spermat(o) | sperm |

After practicing word building and terminology exercises related to the male reproductive system, you will learn about working in a fertility clinic.

## Exercises in the Male Reproductive System

### Building Terms

For each of the following definitions, provide a term using male reproductive system word parts as well as prefixes and suffixes you learned in Units 2 and 3.

1. production of sperm: _____

2. removal of the prostate: _____

3. inflammation of the glans penis: _____

4. resembling sperm: _____

5. herniated testicle: _____

6. lack of sperm: _____

7. inflammation of the prostate and bladder: _____

8. removal of a testicle: _____

9. inflammation of the prostate and seminal vesicles: _____

10. birth control that kills sperm: _____

## Completing Terms

Complete the following terms by adding a prefix or suffix to the word or word part given here.

1. sperm cell: spermato_____

2. inflammation of a testicle: orchid_____

3. scanty amount of sperm: _____spermia

4. plastic surgery on the glans penis: balano_____

5. testicle pain: orchid_____

6. prostate inflammation: prostat_____

7. cyst on the epididymis: spermato_____

8. surgical fixing of a testicle: orchio_____

9. hormone that develops male characteristics: andro_____

10. surgical incision into a testicle: orchido_____

## Finding the Word Parts

Break each of the following terms into words or word parts. Give the definition of the term as well as the meaning of each word or word part.

1. vasovasostomy _____

_____

2. androgen _____

_____

3. orchidocele _____

_____

4. epididymitis: _____

_____

5. prostatovesiculectomy: _____

_____

6. balanoplasty: _____

_____

7. orchidectomy: _____

_____

8. andropathy: _____

_____

9. orchitis: _____

_____

10. spermatogenesis: _____

_____

## Proofreading and Understanding Terms

Write the correct spelling and definition in the blank to the right of any misspelled words. If the spelling is correct, write C.

1. epidymis: _____
2. testosterone: _____
3. spermotazoa: _____
4. testicle: _____
5. vacriocele: _____

6. fimosis: _____
7. circumcision: _____
8. chorde: _____
9. praipism: _____
10. peronie's disease: _____

## Checking Your Work

You have to input information electronically to get insurance reimbursement for a patient. The superbill below has the code, the diagnosis, the patient information, and the dates of service. If the electronic data is not accurate, reimbursement will be withheld. Proofread what you have input and describe any errors you find.

Name _____

Class _____   Date _____

---

Dr. Alan Mirkhan
4567 West Street
New Ridge, AZ 33333
666-333-4444

☐ PRIVATE   ☐ BLUECROSS   ☐ IND.   ☐ MEDICARE   ☐ MEDICAID   ☐ HMO   ☐ PPO

| PATIENT'S LAST NAME | FIRST | ACCOUNT # | BIRTHDATE | SEX ☑ MALE | TODAY'S DATE |
|---|---|---|---|---|---|
| Sweeny | James | X0704 | 01/31/1965 | ☐ FEMALE | 07/08/2010 |

| INSURANCE COMPANY | SUBSCRIBER | PLAN # | SUB. # | GROUP # |
|---|---|---|---|---|
| Healthways, Inc. | | | | |

ASSIGNMENT: I hereby assign my insurance benefits to be paid directly to the undersigned physician. I am financially responsible for non-covered services.
SIGNED: (Patient)
Parent (if Minor)          DATE:   /   /

RELEASE: I hereby authorize the physician to release to my insurance carriers any information requested to process this claim.
SIGNED: (Patient)
Parent (if Minor)          DATE:   /   /

| ✓ | DESCRIPTION | CPT/Med | Dx/Re | PEE | ✓ | DESCRIPTION | CPT/Med | Dx/Re | PEE | ✓ | DESCRIPTION | CPT/Med | Dx/Re | PEE |
|---|---|---|---|---|---|---|---|---|---|---|---|---|---|---|
| | OFFICE CARE | | | | | PROCEDURES | | | | | INJECTIONS/IMMUNIZATIONS | | | |
| | NEW PATIENT | | | | | Treadmill (in Office) | 93015 | | | | Tetanus | | 90718 | |
| | Brief | 99201 | | | | 24-hour Holter | 93224 | | | | Hypertet | J1870 | 90782 | |
| | Limited | 99202 | | | | if Medicare set-up fee | 93225 | | | | Pneumococcal | | 90732 | |
| | Intermediate | 99203 | | | | Physician Interpret | 93227 | | | | Influenza | | 90724 | |
| | Extended | 99204 | | | | EKG w/Interpretation | 93000 | | | | TB Skin Test (PPD) | | 86585 | |
| | Comprehensive | 99205 | | | | EKG (Medicare) | 93005 | | | | Antigen Injection-Single | 95115 | | |
| | | | | | | Sigmoidoscopy | 45300 | | | | Multiple | | 95117 | |
| | ESTABLISHED PATIENT | | | | | Sigmoidoscopy (flexible) | 45330 | | | | B12 Injection | J3420 | 90782 | |
| | Minimal | 99211 | | | | Sigmoidos., Flex. w/Bx. | 45331 | | | | Injection, IM | | 90782 | |
| | Brief | 99212 | | | | Spirometry FEV/FVC | 94010 | | | | Compazine | J0780 | 90782 | |
| | Limited | 99213 | | | | Spirometry, Post-Dilator | 94080 | | | | Demerol | J2175 | 90782 | |
| ✓ | Intermediate | 99214 | | | | | | | | | Vistaril | J3410 | 90782 | |
| | Extended | 99215 | | | | | | | | | Susphrine | J0170 | 90782 | |
| | Comprehensive | 00215 | | | | LABORATORY | | | | | Decadron | J0890 | 90782 | |
| | | | | | ✓ | Blood Draw Fee | 36415 | | | | Estradiol | J1000 | 90782 | |
| | CONSULTATION-OFFICE | | | | | Urinalysis, chemical | 81005 | | | | Testosterone | J1080 | 90782 | |
| | Focused | 99241 | | | | Throat Culture | 87081 | | | | Lidocaine | J2000 | 90782 | |
| | Expanded | 99242 | | | | Occult Blood | 82270 | | | | Solumedrol | J2920 | 90782 | |
| | Detailed | 99243 | | | | Pap Handling Charge | 99000 | | | | Solucortel | J1720 | 90782 | |
| | Comprehensive 1 | 99244 | | | | Pap Life Guard | 88150-90 | | | | Hydeltra | J1680 | 90782 | |
| | Comprehensive 2 | 99245 | | | | Gram Stain | 87205 | | | | Pen Procaine | H2510 | 90788 | |
| | | | | | | Hanging Drop | 87210 | | | | | | | |
| | | | | | | Urine Drug Screen | 99000 | | | | INJECTIONS-JOINT/BURSA | | | |
| | | | | | | | | | | | Small Joints | | 20800 | |
| | | | | | | | | | | | Intermediate | | 20605 | |
| | | | | | | SUPPLIES | | | | | Large Joints | | 20810 | |
| | | | | | | | | | | | Trigger Point | | 20550 | |
| | | | | | | | | | | | MISCELLANEOUS | | | |

| DIAGNOSIS: | ICD-9 | | | | | | | | |
|---|---|---|---|---|---|---|---|---|---|
| __ Abdominal Pain | 789.0 | __ Gout | 274.0 | __ C.V.A. -Acute | 436. | __ Electrolyte Dis. | 276.9 | __ Herpes Simplex | 054.9 |
| __ Abscess (Site) | 682.9 | __ Asthma | 493.90 | __ Cere. Vas. Accid. (Old) | 438 | __ Fatigue | 780.7 | __ Herpes Zoster | 053.9 |
| __ Adverse Drug Rx | 995.2 | __ Asthmatic Bronchitis | 493.90 | __ Cerumen | 380.4 | __ Fibrocys. Br. Dis. | 610.1 | __ Hydrocele | 603.9 |
| __ Alcohol Detox | 291.8 | __ Atrial Fib | 427.31 | __ Chestwall Pain | 786.59 | __ Fracture (Site) | 829.0 | __ Hyperlipidemia | 272.4 |
| __ Alcoholism | 303.90 | __ Atrial Tachi | 427.0 | __ Cholecystitis | 575.0 | __ Open/Close | | __ Hypertension | 401.9 |
| __ Allergic Rhinitis | 477 | __ Bowel Obstruct. | 560.9 | __ Cholelithiasis | 574.00 | __ Fungal Infect. (Site) | 110.8 | __ Hyperthyroidism | 242.9 |
| __ Allergy | 995.3 | __ Breast Mass | 611.72 | __ COPD | 492.8 | __ Gastric Ulcer | 531.90 | __ Hypothyroidism | 244.9 |
| __ Alzheimer's Dis. | 290.1 | __ Bronchitis | 490 | __ Cirrhosis | 571.5 | __ Gastritis | 535.0 | __ Labyrinthitis | 386.30 |
| __ Anemia | 285.9 | __ Bursitis | 727.3 | __ Cong. Heart Fail. | 428.9 | __ Gastroenteritis | 558.9 | __ Lipoma (Site) | 214.9 |
| __ Anemia-Pernicious | 281.0 | __ Cancer, Breast (Site) | 174.9 | __ Conjunctivitis | 372.30 | __ G.I. Bleeding | 578.9 | __ Lymphoma | 202.8 |
| __ Angina | 413.9 | __ Metastatic (Site) | 199.1 | __ Contusion (Site) | 924.9 | __ Glomerulonephritis | 583.9 | __ Mit. Valve Prolapse | 424.0 |
| __ Anxiety Synd. | 300.00 | __ Colon | 153.9 | __ Costochondritis | 733.99 | __ Headache | 784.0 | __ Myocard. Infarction (Area) | 410.9 |
| __ Appendicitis | 541 | __ Cancer, Rectal | 154.1 | __ Depression | 311. | __ Headache, Tension | 307.81 | __ M.I., Old | 412 |
| __ Arteriosci. H.D. | 414.0 | __ Lung (Site) | 162.9 | __ Dermatitis | 692.9 | __ Migrane (Type) | 346.9 | __ Myositis | 729.1 |
| __ Arthritis, Osteo. | 715.90 | __ Skin (Site) | 173.9 | __ Diabetes Mellitus | 250.00 | __ Hemorrhoids | 455.6 | __ Nausea/Vomiting | 767.0 |
| __ Rheumatoid | 714.0 | __ Card. Arrhythmia (Type) | 427.9 | __ Diabetic Ketosis | 250.1 | __ Hernia, Hiatal | 553.3 | __ Neuralgia | 729.2 |
| __ Lupus | 710.0 | __ Cardiomyopathy | 425.4 | __ Diverticulitis | 562.11 | __ Inguinal | 550.9 | __ Nevus (Site) | 216.9 |
| | | __ Cellulitis (Site) | 682.9 | __ Diverticulosis | 562.10 | __ Hepatitis | 573.3 | __ Obesity | 278.0 |

DIAGNOSIS: (IF NOT CHECKED ABOVE)

| SERVICES PERFORMED AT: | ☐ Office | ☐ E.R. | ☐ CLAIM CONTAINS NO ORDERED REFERRING SERVICE | REFERRING PHYSICIAN & I.D. NUMBER |
|---|---|---|---|---|
| ☐ | | ☐ | | |

| RETURN APPOINTMENT INFORMATION: 5 - 10 - 15 - 20 - 30 - 40 - 60 | NEXT APPOINTMENT M - T - W - TH - F - S | | ACCEPT ASSIGNMENT? | DOCTOR'S SIGNATURE |
|---|---|---|---|---|
| [   DAYS] [   WKS.] [   MOS.] [   PRN] | DATE   /   /   TIME: | AM PM | ☐ YES ☐ NO | |

| | | |
|---|---|---|
| ☐ CASH | TOTAL TODAY'S FEE | |
| ☐ CHECK #_____ | OLD BALANCE | |
| ☐ VISA | TOTAL DUE | |
| ☐ MC | | |
| ☐ CO-PAY | AMOUNT REC'D. TODAY | |

1. Complete upper portion of this form, sign and date.
2. Attach this form to your own Insurance company's form for client reimbursement.

MEDICARE PATIENTS - DO NOT SEND THIS TO MEDICARE.
WE WILL SUBMIT THE CLAIM FOR YOU.

Name _____

Class _____ Date _____

---

Patient: John Sweeney          Date: 7/8/2010

Provider: Adan Mirkhan         Visit: New patient visit

Prostate swollen. PSA test taken—will call with results. Schedule follow-up visit in 10 days.

_____

_____

_____

## Filling in the Blanks

1. Sperm is stored in the _____ before being transported to the vas deferens.

2. Semen is expelled during _____.

3. The Cowper's glands are also known as the _____ glands.

4. Erectile tissue is contained within the _____.

5. The area between the anus and the scrotum is the _____.

6. The testes are contained in the _____.

7. Spermatozoa are processed inside the _____.

8. Male sexual characteristics develop during _____.

9. The _____ are glands that secrete testosterone.

10. BPH is benign enlargement of the _____.

## True or False

Circle T for true or F for false.

1. Adolescence begins before puberty.     T     F

2. Oligospermia may be a cause of infertility.     T     F

3. PSA is a test for colon cancer.     T     F

4. Erectile dysfunction is also known as impotence.     T     F

**5.** Phimosis is a congenital condition.    T    F

**6.** STDs can be transmitted by both males and females.    T    F

**7.** A digital rectal exam tests for prostate enlargement.    T    F

**8.** An orchiectomy removes a diseased prostate.    T    F

**9.** A vasectomy is a form of male birth control.    T    F

**10.** Infertility is affected by the motility of sperm.    T    F

## Using a Dictionary

Using your allied health dictionary, define the purpose of the following male hormones.

**1.** testosterone: _____

_____

**2.** androsterone: _____

_____

**3.** follicle-stimulating hormone (FSH): _____

_____

**4.** luteinizing hormone (LH): _____

_____

**5.** inhibin: _____

_____

## Writing the Medical Term

For each of the following descriptions, write the proper medical term or an alternative medical term.

**1.** undescended testicle: _____

**7.** tail of a sperm: _____

**2.** sexual intercourse: _____

**8.** development of sperm: _____

**3.** impotence: _____

**9.** head of the penis _____

**4.** testicular tumor: _____

**10.** expulsion of semen outside the body: _____

**5.** male sex glands: _____

**6.** foreskin: _____

## Word Find

In the following puzzle, draw a line around at least 20 words pertaining to the integumentary system. The words can be horizontal, vertical, diagonal, or upside-down. Write the words on the rules provided. If you do not know the meaning of a word, look it up in your allied health dictionary and make a flash card for future review.

| a | r | g | h | r | w | v | b | n | h | y | a | b | e | g | h | j | h | b | s |
|---|---|---|---|---|---|---|---|---|---|---|---|---|---|---|---|---|---|---|---|
| w | n | q | b | n | x | v | b | n | h | j | a | r | t | y | u | a | y | x | t |
| m | h | a | q | w | g | t | n | h | j | l | n | m | h | a | t | p | d | e | e |
| r | y | s | b | c | h | e | u | n | a | f | g | y | i | j | j | r | r | n | s |
| e | p | b | m | o | k | s | k | n | d | v | t | n | e | k | l | i | o | o | t |
| p | o | b | n | k | l | t | t | t | f | c | r | m | e | e | s | a | c | r | i |
| s | s | v | c | n | j | i | t | k | l | e | e | v | n | m | d | p | e | e | c |
| l | p | j | a | o | s | s | c | p | h | i | p | s | n | m | e | i | l | t | l |
| w | a | s | a | s | y | t | n | s | b | k | i | i | h | y | d | s | e | s | e |
| c | d | p | x | c | d | s | e | m | t | k | l | r | s | e | b | m | n | o | w |
| x | i | r | n | e | u | e | k | l | m | e | e | y | v | p | u | i | j | t | l |
| a | a | o | w | n | m | l | f | s | r | y | r | j | k | l | a | e | c | s | e |
| s | s | s | c | n | p | m | a | r | w | j | k | o | n | i | t | d | s | e | m |
| p | y | t | h | a | h | b | e | t | e | s | a | v | i | g | j | q | i | t | c |
| e | m | a | a | n | i | b | m | k | i | n | a | q | t | d | j | o | p | a | b |
| r | o | t | n | w | m | v | w | n | e | o | s | r | n | k | s | s | s | q | s |
| m | t | i | c | h | o | j | e | l | o | p | n | x | j | m | l | t | w | y | h |
| i | c | s | r | i | s | p | j | d | z | e | r | h | i | o | r | g | v | n | m |
| a | e | z | o | n | i | i | p | m | u | l | l | e | g | a | l | f | m | u | l |
| a | s | w | i | q | s | n | m | x | i | p | g | w | t | k | v | e | t | m | p |
| u | a | i | d | k | i | m | q | m | u | e | n | i | r | e | p | o | c | r | r |
| j | v | i | s | p | l | a | n | t | m | q | o | v | e | k | r | a | h | i | o |
| m | e | c | h | b | y | u | i | o | l | n | b | x | m | c | j | i | l | p | s |
| i | n | f | e | r | t | i | l | i | t | y | x | z | s | w | b | n | i | j | t |
| c | r | w | n | y | u | i | o | p | l | e | c | n | e | t | o | p | m | i | a |
| x | c | i | r | c | u | m | s | i | c | i | o | n | k | o | p | r | w | c | t |
| g | l | a | n | s | p | e | n | i | s | a | a | m | o | n | i | m | e | s | e |
| j | i | n | x | u | l | e | p | i | d | i | d | y | m | i | s | a | w | r | n |

a. _____          n. _____

b. _____          o. _____

c. _____          p. _____

d. _____          q. _____

e. _____          r. _____

f. _____          s. _____

g. _____          t. _____

h. _____          u. _____

i. _____          v. _____

j. _____          w. _____

k. _____          x. _____

l. _____          y. _____

m. _____          z. _____

## Working in a Clinic

Jose Aguilerez is a medical assistant in a male infertility clinic. His duties range from scheduling appointments to dealing with patients both as they arrive and as they are escorted to examination rooms. Because this is a small clinic located in a medical building, Jose is the only worker besides the doctor and a part-time billing clerk. Because his duties are so varied, Jose has had to learn many skills.

## Using a Scheduler

The clinic uses a computerized scheduling system. Jose works Tuesdays through Saturdays from 10–6 with late hours on Thursday until 9. Patients are seen every day from 10–3 with an hour for lunch from 12–1.

Schedule appointments for the following five patients:
**M. Carlson**: can only come after work (he finishes at 4:30 every day) or on Saturday.
**J. Allegro**: works second shift and can come almost any time until 3:00 but not on Saturday.
**L. Smith**: is a college professor and will be on break for the next two weeks.
**T. Baxter**: can come in only on Saturdays or Thursday after 6.
**J. Velez**: works every day but Tuesday.

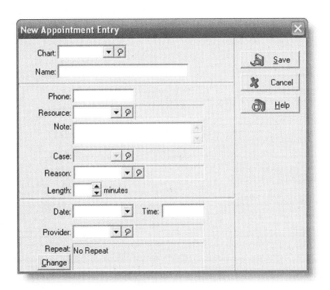

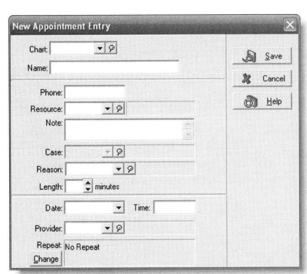

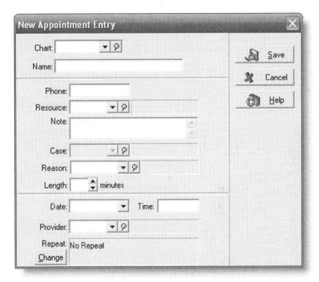

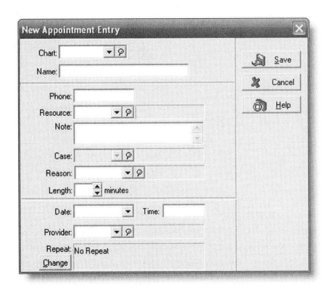

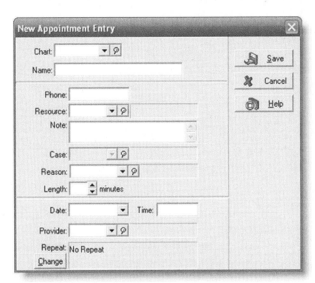

Make calls to the five patients above. Describe each call. Either leave a message asking each one to confirm the appointment or speak to the person if he or she answers.

1. _____
   _____
   _____

2. _____
   _____
   _____

3. _____
   _____
   _____

4. _____
   _____
   _____

5. _____
   _____
   _____

# UNIT 12

# Terms in the Blood System

## Word Parts in the Blood System

These are the major word parts used to form words in the blood system. When you combine these parts with some of the prefixes and suffixes in Units 2 and 3, you will be able to understand medical terms relating to the blood system.

| | |
|---|---|
| agglutin(o) | agglutinin |
| erythr(o) | red |
| hemo, hemat(o) | blood |
| leuk(o) | white |
| phag(o) | eating, devouring |
| thromb(o) | blood clot |

After practicing word building and terminology exercises related to the blood system, you will learn about working as a laboratory technician.

## Exercises in the Blood System

### Building Terms

For each of the following definitions, provide a term using blood system word parts as well as prefixes and suffixes you learned in Units 2 and 3.

1. immature red blood cell: _____

2. blood in the urine: _____

3. formation of white blood cells: _____

4. cell that devours other cells: _____

5. blood specialist: _____

6. immature white blood cell: _____

7. mature red blood cell: _____

**8.** blood in the feces: _____

**9.** stopping of bleeding: _____

**10.** cancer of the blood: _____

## Completing Terms

Complete the following terms by adding a prefix or suffix to the word or word part given here.

**1.** agent that causes agglutinin to form: agglutino_____

**2.** red blood cell production in bone marrow: erythro_____

**3.** decreased numbers of all types of blood cells: _____cytopenia

**4.** within a blood vessel: _____vascular

**5.** vomiting of blood: hemat_____

**6.** condition of low number of white blood cells: leukocyt_____

**7.** formation of blood cells: hemato_____

**8.** excessive bleeding: hemo_____

**9.** substance that comes before a thrombus: _____thrombin

**10.** disease without enough red blood cells: _____emia

## Finding the Word Parts

Break each of the following terms into words or word parts. Give the definition of the term as well as the meaning of each word or word part.

**1.** erythroleukemia: _____

_____

**2.** hemarthrosis: _____

_____

**3.** hematocyte: __ _____

_____ _____

**4.** erythrocytopenia: _____

_____

**5.** hemoptysis: _____

_____

**6.** erythrocyanosis: _____

_____

**7.** hemodialysis: _____

_____

**8.** hemothorax: _____

_____

**9.** phagocytosis: _____

_____

**10.** polycythemia: _____

_____

## Proofreading and Understanding Terms

Write the correct spelling and definition in the blank to the right of any misspelled words. If the spelling is correct, write C.

**1.** erythropoieitin: _____

**2.** nutrophil: _____

**3.** platelet: _____

**4.** basophil: _____

**5.** eosinophil: _____

**6.** agranlocyte: _____

**7.** thalasemia: _____

**8.** venapuncture: _____

**9.** hemolisis: _____

**10.** embolus: _____

The CBC shown below has some spelling errors. Describe what you find.

| | | | |
|---|---|---|---|
| Elyse Armadian, M.D.<br>3 South Windsor Street<br>Fairfield, MN 00219<br>300-546-7890 | Laboratory Report<br>Sunview Diagnostics<br>6712 Adams Drive<br>Fairfield, MN 00220<br>300-546-7000 | | |

| | | |
|---|---|---|
| Patient: Janine Josephs | Patient ID: 099-00-1200 | Date of Birth: 08/07/43 |
| Date Collected: 09/30/XXXX | Time Collected: 16:05 | Total Volume: 2000 |
| Date Received: 09/30/XXXX | Date Reported: 10/06/XXXX | |

| Test | Result | Flag | Reference |
|---|---|---|---|
| *Complete Blood Count* | | | |
| WBD | 4.0 | | 3.9-11.1 |
| RBC | 4.11 | | 3.80-5.20 |
| HCT | 39.7 | | 34.0-47.0 |
| MCV | 96.5 | | 80.0-98.0 |
| MCH | 32.9 | | 27.1-34.0 |
| MCHC | 34.0 | | 32.0-36.0 |
| MPV | 8.6 | | 7.5-11.5 |
| NEUTROPHILS % | 45.6 | | 38.0-80.0 |
| NEUTROPHILS ABS. | 1.82 | | 1.70-8.50 |
| LYMPHOCYTES % | 36.1 | | 15.0-49.0 |
| LYMPHOCYTES ABS. | 1.44 | | 1.00-3.50 |
| ESINOPHILS % | 4.5 | | 0.0-8.0 |
| ESINOPHILS ABS. | 0.18 | | 0.03-0.55 |
| BASOPHILS % | 0.7 | | 0.0-2.0 |
| BASOPHILS ABS. | 0.03 | | 0.000-0.185 |
| PLATLET COUNT | 229 | | 150-400 |
| | | | |
| *Automated Chemistries* | | | |
| GLUCOSE | 80 | | 65-109 |
| UREA NITROGEN | 17 | | 6-30 |
| CREATININE (SERUM) | 0.6 | | 0.5-1.3 |
| UREA NITROGEN/CREATININE | 28 | | 10-29 |
| SODIUM | 140 | | 135-145 |
| POTASSIUM | 4.4 | | 3.5-5.3 |
| CHLORIDE | 106 | | 96-109 |
| $CO_2$ | 28 | | 20-31 |
| ANION GAP | 6 | | 3-19 |
| CALCIUM | 9.8 | | 8.6-10.4 |
| PHOSPHORUS | 3.6 | | 2.2-4.6 |
| AST (SGOT) | 28 | | 0-30 |
| ALT (SGPT) | 19 | | 0-34 |
| BILIRUBIN, TOTAL | 0.5 | | 0.2-1.2 |
| PROTEIN, TOTAL | 7.8 | | 6.2-8.2 |
| ALBUMIN | 4.3 | | 3.5-5.0 |
| GLOBULIN | 3.5 | | 2.1-3.8 |
| URIC ACID | 2.4 | | 2.0-7.5 |
| CHOLESTEROL | 232 | * | 120-199 |
| TRIGLYCERIDES | 68 | | 40-199 |
| IRON | 85 | | 30-150 |
| HDL CHOLESTEROL | 73 | * | 35-59 |
| CHOLESTEROL/HDL RATIO | 3.2 | | 3.2-5.7 |
| LDL, CALCULATED | 148 | * | 70-129 |
| T3, UPTAKE | 32 | | 24-37 |
| T4, TOTAL | 6.9 | | 4.5-12.8 |

_____

_____

_____

_____

## Filling In the Blanks

1. The clear portion of the blood that carries blood cells and other substances is _____.

2. The process of clotting is _____.

3. The percentage of red blood cells is determined in a(n) _____.

4. Donor blood is given in a(n) _____.

5. A(n) _____ is trained to draw blood.

6. A blood clot that moves is a(n) _____.

7. Small pinpoint hemorrhages are _____.

8. A CBC is a common type of _____ test.

9. Agent that prevents blood clots is a(n) _____.

10. Plasma is separated from the blood cells in _____.

## True or False

Circle T for true or F for false.

1. An eosinophil is a type of red blood cell.    T    F

2. Type A blood contains type A antigens.    T    F

3. A thrombus usually precedes hemorrhaging.    T    F

4. Hemophiliacs lack clotting factor.    T    F

5. Erythropoietin is produced in the spleen.    T    F

6. Sickle cell anemia is an inherited disease.    T    F

7. Erythrocyte is another name for a mature red blood cell.    T    F

8. White blood cells only appear in certain diseases.    T    F

9. Anisocytosis is a condition with excessive inequality in size of red blood cells.     T     F

10. Hematologist is another name for a phlebotomist.     T     F

## Using a Dictionary

Using your allied health dictionary, look up the following abbreviations. Write out what they are abbreviating and give a brief definition of each.

1. CBC: _____

2. ESR: _____

3. Hgb: _____

4. MCV: _____

5. WBC: _____

6. HCT: _____

7. PLT: _____

8. RBC: _____

9. PTT: _____

10. PT: _____

## Writing the Medical Term

For each of the following descriptions, write the proper medical term or an alternative medical term.

1. blood cancer: _____

2. tired blood: _____

3. annual blood test: _____

4. blood clot: _____

5. blood thinner: _____

Name _____

Class _____ Date _____

## Word Find

In the following puzzle, draw a line around at least 20 words pertaining to the integumentary system. The words can be horizontal, vertical, diagonal, or upside-down. Write the words on the rules provided. If you do not know the meaning of a word, look it up in your allied health dictionary and make a flash card for future review.

| x | y | l | e | c | h | j | c | m | b | f | i | b | r | i | n | o | g | e | n |
|---|---|---|---|---|---|---|---|---|---|---|---|---|---|---|---|---|---|---|---|
| a | b | s | l | m | k | l | o | o | x | y | n | q | y | g | e | n | j | l | k |
| a | r | n | j | e | i | r | h | f | a | c | t | o | r | v | t | r | m | k | l |
| a | i | c | a | r | c | s | y | d | o | g | x | f | w | r | y | h | k | l | q |
| m | b | l | o | o | d | d | k | u | i | d | u | x | g | n | c | e | t | j | k |
| e | g | n | k | l | u | o | o | a | m | s | a | l | p | z | o | g | n | w | y |
| p | u | r | p | u | r | a | n | o | j | k | o | e | a | b | r | m | a | l | r |
| x | t | a | w | j | k | e | k | l | l | b | t | h | x | n | h | s | l | d | e |
| d | b | y | n | w | m | c | d | d | i | b | s | o | m | k | t | u | u | e | d |
| x | a | g | n | e | k | t | d | n | w | q | e | t | i | u | y | y | g | o | b |
| r | i | t | h | u | m | e | y | n | j | k | c | t | e | y | r | k | a | l | l |
| e | n | c | n | j | k | i | w | e | l | v | b | r | i | w | e | f | o | k | o |
| l | e | u | k | e | m | i | a | m | k | s | u | i | l | h | s | w | c | b | o |
| a | p | t | y | k | l | m | w | x | t | t | y | j | k | m | w | o | i | q | d |
| p | o | n | k | e | f | g | h | j | l | e | n | k | e | w | c | m | t | l | c |
| s | r | z | n | f | e | q | u | u | e | m | u | y | n | i | t | x | n | u | e |
| e | h | k | i | l | u | i | c | l | q | c | e | b | n | i | l | n | a | e | l |
| x | t | t | m | m | k | d | u | m | y | e | l | o | b | l | a | s | t | v | l |
| x | y | n | u | w | o | e | m | d | t | l | y | l | q | v | m | z | r | t | h |
| l | r | q | b | o | w | y | j | c | s | l | w | h | i | o | l | p | b | n | m |
| e | e | t | l | m | u | l | s | c | i | e | t | h | e | m | o | l | p | w | x |
| b | h | b | a | n | m | u | i | i | s | w | x | m | k | p | k | l | l | m | a |
| d | g | r | a | n | u | l | o | c | y | t | e | j | l | d | a | w | u | x | m |
| m | k | r | v | t | i | m | k | o | l | p | s | c | m | e | t | r | j | o | p |
| e | o | s | i | n | o | b | a | s | o | p | h | i | l | v | e | m | i | m | y |
| a | v | m | k | u | i | e | x | u | m | r | e | m | i | s | s | i | o | n | l |
| t | e | l | e | t | a | l | p | x | e | w | y | u | n | d | s | a | z | y | b |
| e | b | h | j | k | l | w | q | z | h | i | s | t | a | m | i | n | e | e | z |

a. _____     e. _____

b. _____     f. _____

c. _____     g. _____

d. _____     h. _____

i. _____        r. _____

j. _____        s. _____

k. _____        t. _____

l. _____        u. _____

m. _____        v. _____

n. _____        w. _____

o. _____        x. _____

p. _____        y. _____

q. _____        z. _____

## Working as a Lab Technician

You are a lab technician and are trained as a phlebotomist. You work in a small medical laboratory where you take the blood and urine samples from clients and do the processing.

## Taking Samples

The first client of the day hands in the form on page 143. What samples will you be taking?

_____

_____

_____

_____

## Reading Lab Results

The CBC report on page 144 showed some abnormal readings. Which tests showed abnormal readings?

_____

_____

_____

_____

Name _____

Class _____ Date _____

---

**Archway Diagnostics**
75 Main Street
Weldon, OK 77788
666-666-6666

| FAC CODE | DATE | TIME COLLECTED | LABORATORY USE ONLY |
|---|---|---|---|
| | | : AM | |
| DRAWN BY | | : PM | |

### CLIENT

Susan Mayberry, MD
8420 Independence Ave.
Alton, AL 66666
888-999-7777

**PATIENT INFORMATION**

| NAME (LAST, FIRST, MIDDLE, INITIAL) | PATIENT ID NO. |
|---|---|
| ALVARNEY, JANE | 077-777-7777 |

| ADDRESS |
|---|
| 14 Ashway Dr. |

| CITY | STATE | ZIPCODE | MALE | FEMALE | DATE OF BIRTH |
|---|---|---|---|---|---|
| Alton | AL | 66661 | ☐ | ☑ | 06/14/86 |

| ICD CODE (REQUIRED) | SYSMPTOM | PATIENT TELEPHONE NO |
|---|---|---|

PHYSICIAN IF DIFFERENT/REPORTING REMARKS
☐ FASTING
☐ NON-FASTING

PLEASE BILL TO: ☐ PATIENT BILL ☑ CLIENT/DOCTOR ☐ INSURANCE

REPORTING COMMENTS:

**PRIMARY INSURANCE**

| INSURANCE NAME | STATE | INSURED'S NAME |
|---|---|---|

CARBON COPY TO:
(CLIENT CODE OR FULL NAME AND FULL ADDRESS w. ZIP CODE)

| RELATIONSHIP TO PATIENT | PATIENT'S (OR INSURED'S) I.D. NUMBER |
|---|---|
| ☐ SELF ☐ SPOUSE ☐ CHILD ☐ OTHER | |

| GROUP NO. | INSURED'S EMPLOYER | PAYOR NUMBER |
|---|---|---|

**SECONDARY INSURANCE**

| INSURANCE NAME | STATE | INSURED'S NAME |
|---|---|---|

☐ STAT & CALL
☐ CALL RESULT
☐ FAX

TELEPHONE NUMBER
( )
FAX NUMBER
( )

| RELATIONSHIP TO PATIENT | PATIENT'S (OR INSURED'S) I.D. NUMBER |
|---|---|
| ☐ SELF ☐ SPOUSE ☐ CHILD ☐ OTHER | |

| GROUP NO. | INSURED'S EMPLOYER | PAYOR NUMBER |
|---|---|---|

URINE COLLECTION VOLUME
☐ 24 HOURS
☐ RANDOM
_____ ML: ☐ _____ HRS:

TECHNICAL NOTES:

I authorize Archway Diagnostics to release information received, including without limitation, medical information, which includes laboratory test results to my health plan/insurance carrier, and its authorized representatives, I further authorize my health plan/insurance carrier to directly pay Quest Diagnostics for the service rendered.

PATIENT SIGNATURE :

| LABORATORY USE ONLY | 98242 | BLOOD DRAWING FEE | 98245 | HANDLING | 98253 | HOUSE CALL-PVT | 98371 | SINGLE PATIENT-NH | 98372 | MULTI PATIENT-NH |
|---|---|---|---|---|---|---|---|---|---|---|

| CHEMISTRY TESTS | PANELS/PROFILES | OTHER TESTS | OTHER TESTS |
|---|---|---|---|
| X1234 ☐ Albumin | 226 ☐ Electrolyte Panel | 5647 ☐ Amylase | 4111 ☐ Lyme screen |
| X1233 ☐ Alkaline phosph. | 777 ☐ Lipid Panel | 4333 ☐ Blood group and Rh | 6665 ☐ Progesterone |
| X1245 ☐ ALT (SGPT) | 888 ☐ Metabolic Panel | 6767 ☐ CA-125 | 7676 ☐ Prothrombin time |
| V1222 ☐ AST (SGOT) | 666 ☐ Lipid Panel | 8888 ☐ C-Reactive protein | 8111 ☐ PSA |
| V1234 ☐ Bilirubin, Total | **PROFILES** | 5555 ☑ CBC | 9988 ☐ Testosterone |
| Y3333 ☐ Calcium | 456 ☐ Hepatitis Profiles | 5555A ☐ CBC w/diff | 7676 ☑ Urinalysis complete |
| Y1234 ☐ Carbon Dioxide | 998 ☐ Obstetric Panel | 6789 ☐ Digoxin | 8866 ☐ Vit B12 |
| Y4354 ☐ Chloride | **MICROBIOLOGY** | 7890 ☐ Dilantin | |
| M5555 ☐ Cholesterol | 009 ☐ Chlamydia | 6543 ☐ Estradiol | |
| P6666 ☐ Creatinine | 437 ☐ Gonorrhea | 7776 ☐ Folate | |
| M0099 ☐ Glucose | **Cultures:** | 1221 ☐ FSH | |
| L6565 ☐ Iron | 990 ☐ Blood | 1117 ☐ H. Pylori | |
| Y7777 ☐ Magnesium | 888 ☐ Ear | 2223 ☐ HCG | |
| P0000 ☐ Phosphorus | 777 ☐ Eye | 5556 ☐ HDL | |
| Y3456 ☐ Protein, total | 444 ☐ Genital | 7778 ☐ HIV–W. blot | |
| U7890 ☐ Sodium | 333 ☑ Sputum | 8885 ☐ Herpes | |
| W2345 ☐ Triglycerides | 787 ☐ Stool | 3334 ☐ Iron | |
| Z3456 ☐ Urea nitrogen | | 6667 ☐ Lead | |
| H5555 ☐ Uric acid | | 8787 ☐ LH & FSH | |

*Source:*
OTHER TESTS:

_____
AUTHORISING PHYSICIAN SIGNATURE

You process a CBC and the computer prints out the following results.

| Thomas Chen, M.D.<br>16 Waterview Rd.<br>Andala, CA 55555<br>306-000-9999 | Laboratory Report<br>Sunview Diagnostics<br>6712 Adams Drive<br>Fairfield, MN 00220<br>300-546-7000 | |
|---|---|---|
| Patient: John Rudy<br>Date Collected: 09/30/XXXX<br>Date Received: 09/30/XXXX | Patient ID: 099-00-1200<br>Time Collected: 16:05<br>Date Reported: 10/06/XXXX | Date of Birth: 08/07/57<br>Total Volume: 2000 |

| Test | Result | Flag | Reference |
|---|---|---|---|
| *Complete Blood Count* | | | |
| WBC | 4.0 | | 3.9-11.1 |
| RBC | 4.11 | | 3.80-5.20 |
| HCT | 39.7 | | 34.0-47.0 |
| MCV | 96.5 | | 80.0-98.0 |
| MCH | 32.9 | | 27.1-34.0 |
| MCHC | 34.0 | | 32.0-36.0 |
| MPV | 8.6 | | 7.5-11.5 |
| NEUTROPHILS % | 45.6 | | 38.0-80.0 |
| NEUTROPHILS ABS. | 1.82 | | 1.70-8.50 |
| LYMPHOCYTES % | 36.1 | | 15.0-49.0 |
| LYMPHOCYTES ABS. | 1.44 | | 1.00-3.50 |
| EOSINOPHILS % | 4.5 | | 0.0-8.0 |
| EOSINOPHILS ABS. | 0.18 | | 0.03-0.55 |
| BASOPHILS % | 0.7 | | 0.0-2.0 |
| BASOPHILS ABS. | 0.03 | | 0.000-0.185 |
| PLATELET COUNT | 450 | * | 150-400 |
| | | | |
| *Automated Chemistries* | | | |
| GLUCOSE | 80 | | 65-109 |
| UREA NITROGEN | 17 | | 6-30 |
| CREATININE (SERUM) | 0.6 | | 0.5-1.3 |
| UREA NITROGEN/CREATININE | 28 | | 10-29 |
| SODIUM | 140 | | 135-145 |
| POTASSIUM | 4.4 | * | 3.5-5.3 |
| CHLORIDE | 106 | | 96-109 |
| $CO_2$ | 28 | | 20-31 |
| ANION GAP | 6 | | 3-19 |
| CALCIUM | 9.8 | | 8.6-10.4 |
| PHOSPHORUS | 3.6 | | 2.2-4.6 |
| AST (SGOT) | 28 | | 0-30 |
| ALT (SGPT) | 19 | | 0-34 |
| BILIRUBIN, TOTAL | 0.5 | | 0.2-1.2 |
| PROTEIN, TOTAL | 7.8 | | 6.2-8.2 |
| ALBUMIN | 4.3 | | 3.5-5.0 |
| GLOBULIN | 3.5 | | 2.1-3.8 |
| URIC ACID | 2.4 | | 2.0-7.5 |
| CHOLESTEROL | 232 | * | 120-199 |
| TRIGLYCERIDES | 68 | | 40-199 |
| IRON | 85 | | 30-150 |
| HDL CHOLESTEROL | 73 | * | 35-59 |
| CHOLESTEROL/HDL RATIO | 3.2 | | 3.2-5.7 |
| LDL, CALCULATED | 148 | * | 70-129 |
| T3, UPTAKE | 32 | | 24-37 |
| T4, TOTAL | 6.9 | | 4.5-12.8 |

# Terms in the Lymphatic and Immune System

## Word Parts in the Lymphatic and Immune Systems

These are the major word parts used to form words in the lymphatic and immune systems. When you combine these parts with some of the prefixes and suffixes in Units 2 and 3, you will be able to understand medical terms relating to the lymphatic and immune systems.

| | |
|---|---|
| aden(o) | gland |
| immun(o) | immunity |
| lymph(o) | lymph |
| lymphaden(o) | lymph nodes |
| lymphangi(o) | lymphatic vessels |
| splen(o) | spleen |
| thym(o) | thymus |
| tox(o), toxi, toxico | poison |

After practicing word building and terminology exercises related to the lymphatic and immune systems, you will learn about working in a medical clinic.

## Exercises in the Lymphatic and Immune Systems

### Building Terms

For each of the following definitions, provide a term using lymphatic and immune system word parts as well as prefixes and suffixes you learned in Units 2 and 3.

1. glandular inflammation: _____

2. spleen hemorrhage: _____

3. agent that depresses the immune system: _____

4. surgical removal of a lymph node: _____

5. glandular pain: _____

6. enlargement of the spleen: _____

7. having reduced immunity: _____

8. removal of a spleen: _____

9. inflammation of lymph vessels: _____

10. science of the relationship between immunity and genetics: _____

11. proteins that function as antibodies in immunity: _____

12. inflammation of lymph nodes resulting from infection: _____

13. swelling caused by an accumulation of lymph: _____

14. suture of a ruptured spleen: _____

15. benign tumor of the thymus: _____

## Completing Terms

Complete the following terms by adding a prefix or suffix to the word or word part given here.

1. disease of the lymph nodes: adeno_____

2. of the spleen: splen_____

3. disease caused by poisoning: toxi_____

4. able to have an immune response: immuno_____

5. primary lymph cell: lympho_____

6. spleen inflammation: splen_____

7. specialist in the immune system: immuno_____

8. blockage of lymph flow: lympho_____

9. surgical removal of the thymus: thym_____

10. study of the effects of poison: toxico_____

11. treatment by triggering the immune system: immuno_____

12. lymphatic tumor: lymph_____

**13.** impaired immunity: immuno_____

**14.** immature lymph cell: lympho_____

**15.** disease of the spleen: spleno_____

## Finding the Word Parts

Break each of the following terms into words or word parts. Give the definition of the term as well as the meaning of each word or word part.

**1.** immunosuppression: _____

_____

**2.** toxicology: _____

_____

**3.** antiretroviral: _____

_____

**4.** cytotoxic: _____

_____

**5.** lymphocytosis: _____

_____

**6.** lymphoma: _____

_____

**7.** lymphadenography: _____

_____

**8.** toxicosis: _____

_____

**9.** cytoplasm: _____

_____

**10.** monocyte: _____

_____

## Proofreading and Understanding Terms

Write the correct spelling and definition in the blank to the right of any misspelled words. If the spelling is correct, write C.

1. limphosarcoma: _____

2. intraferon: _____

3. antebody: _____

4. immunity: _____

5. lymphocite: _____

6. hipersenstivity: _____

7. anaphilasis: _____

8. histamines: _____

9. imunosuppressant: _____

10. Karpasi's sarcoma: _____

The following referral letter describes allergy symptoms to a specialist. Proofread the letter and make two lists, one of the spelling errors (with correction) and one of words that relate to the immune system.

Allen J. Madsen, MD
41 Indian Trail Way
Madison, WI 88888
666-777-9999

Dear Dr. Williams:

Your office has an appointment schedule for a Leila Jonas, a patient of mine. Leila has multiple sclerosis which has been progressing slowly since diagnosis 10 years ago. From time to time, she experiences mild allergies but recently had a case of anafilaxis and was treated in the emergency room. I suspected a reaction to seafood but would like you to do a complete allergy work-up so we can avoid emergencies in the future. I am enclosing her most recent lab tests as well as a list of her current medications. I would be happy to work with on a corse of treatment for this pantient.

Sincerely yours,

*Allen Madsen*

Allen Madsen

Spelling errors:

_____

_____

_____

_____

_____

Words relating to the immune system:

_____

_____

_____

_____

_____

## Filling In the Blanks

1. Monocytes become _____.

2. The _____ response helps the body fight infections.

3. The virus that causes AIDs is abbreviated _____.

4. The largest organ of the lymphatic system is the _____.

5. Organisms that cause disease are called _____.

6. AIDS patients often contract _____ infections.

7. In response to microorganisms, the body releases _____.

8. B cells activate helper _____ cells.

9. A mother provides _____ immunity to her baby.

10. Immunoglobulins are types of _____.

11. AIDS is primarily transmitted _____.

12. Hodgkin's disease is a type of _____.

13. Multiple sclerosis is a type of _____ disease.

14. The release of histamine occurs during a(n) _____ reaction.

15. ELISA is a test for _____.

## True or False

Circle T for true or F for false.

1. You can contract AIDS via airborne particles.     T     F

2. Allergies are infectious.     T     F

3. Vaccines can provide immunity.     T     F

4. Anaphylaxis is a mild allergic reaction.     T     F

5. DPT is a vaccine against allergies.     T     F

6. Rheumatoid arthritis is not an autoimmune disease.     T     F

7. The thymus is more important in little children than in adults.     T     F

8. Some diseases have been virtually eradicated through the use of vaccines.     T     F

9. Swollen lymph nodes are one sign of mononucleosis.     T     F

10. Scleroderma is a highly contagious disease.     T     F

## Using a Dictionary

Using your allied health dictionary, define the following types of immunity.

1. natural immunity: _____

_____

_____

2. passive immunity: _____

_____

_____

3. active immunity: _____

_____

_____

4. acquired immunity: _____

_____

_____

5. acquired active immunity: _____

_____

_____

## Writing the Medical Term

For each of the following descriptions, write the proper medical term or an alternative medical term.

1. extreme allergic reaction: _____

2. childhood shots: _____

3. AIDS virus: _____

4. AIDS pneumonia: _____

Name _____

Class _____ Date _____

## Word Find

In the following puzzle, draw a line around at least 20 words pertaining to the integumentary system. The words can be horizontal, vertical, diagonal, or upside-down. Write the words on the rules provided. If you do not know the meaning of a word, look it up in your allied health dictionary and make a flash card for future review.

| p | h | a | g | o | c | y | t | o | s | i | s | y | s | i | s | n | m | j | w |
|---|---|---|---|---|---|---|---|---|---|---|---|---|---|---|---|---|---|---|---|
| a | n | t | i | c | h | i | s | n | h | m | a | w | d | t | h | k | l | i | o |
| c | d | n | a | l | g | s | u | m | y | h | t | n | t | o | p | c | o | e | n |
| b | n | n | c | t | e | r | r | o | m | i | n | a | h | d | b | j | l | k | l |
| b | w | e | a | x | s | d | i | a | h | l | n | v | y | c | e | i | w | a | k |
| i | o | g | o | c | y | t | v | e | n | t | a | t | m | k | s | l | t | w | a |
| t | l | o | v | x | a | t | o | n | k | o | l | p | e | a | s | s | e | n | z |
| n | i | h | q | n | m | t | r | e | s | x | k | j | c | r | c | l | x | a | a |
| s | a | t | n | m | o | n | t | d | p | i | b | m | t | j | f | l | l | q | a |
| p | l | a | s | m | a | c | e | l | l | c | n | y | o | k | z | e | m | k | l |
| l | w | p | h | m | s | y | r | q | e | o | m | l | m | i | l | c | r | d | c |
| e | i | m | m | u | n | i | t | y | e | s | b | y | y | n | k | b | i | o | e |
| n | m | k | l | e | d | a | v | n | n | i | n | l | m | e | y | l | j | i | n |
| e | l | x | z | a | n | e | i | t | k | s | i | y | l | n | m | k | s | y | e |
| c | y | n | k | v | t | c | w | u | i | l | y | m | p | h | n | o | d | e | j |
| t | m | w | q | m | c | k | y | q | c | n | i | p | m | e | i | d | y | w | j |
| o | p | l | j | a | e | s | t | g | n | c | c | h | o | l | s | n | m | t | y |
| m | h | x | v | v | y | j | h | k | r | m | w | o | c | p | o | t | h | h | k |
| y | o | v | e | y | m | n | y | o | d | e | w | m | q | e | m | n | s | y | l |
| i | c | a | w | c | e | k | p | x | c | w | l | a | q | r | y | i | o | m | l |
| b | y | b | v | y | t | h | a | s | n | k | t | l | h | c | h | l | m | o | n |
| x | t | c | b | r | a | h | m | u | u | i | k | l | a | e | t | a | x | m | n |
| s | e | n | t | g | s | s | m | p | y | j | s | s | h | l | l | q | b | a | y |
| m | s | k | e | l | t | s | d | u | w | q | n | k | l | l | l | o | n | b | v |
| e | b | n | m | r | a | l | u | l | l | e | c | y | a | l | a | g | t | r | m |
| c | u | g | n | e | s | s | f | h | k | e | m | u | p | l | e | k | a | b | m |
| n | i | x | o | t | i | t | n | a | i | p | w | d | h | g | s | c | m | k | q |
| a | k | l | r | o | s | p | k | l | h | u | m | o | r | a | l | q | t | c | m |

a. _____     e. _____

b. _____     f. _____

c. _____     g. _____

d. _____     h. _____

i. _____        r. _____

j. _____        s. _____

k. _____        t. _____

l. _____        u. _____

m. _____        v. _____

n. _____        w. _____

o. _____        x. _____

p. _____        y. _____

q. _____        z. _____

## Working in a Medical Clinic

You are a receptionist in a medical clinic that serves an area of a large city. Most of the clients are on Medicaid or Medicare. The waiting room is always crowded and you often have to handle people who have had to wait for a long time.

## Maintaining Order

As receptionist, it is your job to greet all clients, put them on a list in order as they arrive, get charts for old clients, and set up new patient information for new clients, and check all insurance cards. Since privacy is a prime concern, you ask each client to sign in and then wait to be called. You call each person in to the small enclosed reception area where you can talk to them.

The first client is elderly and seems somewhat disoriented. Ask her to come in to the reception area and describe how you would try to get the information you need to get her help.

_____

_____

_____

_____

_____

The next client is new. His address is 16 Walker St., Abilene, KS 77777; His phone is 888-777-9999. You ask for the insurance card and you enter the new patient into the computer. You photocopy the card. Enter the patient's information into the computer screen.

Greenway Health, Inc.
www.greenway.com
Name(s)

Munoz, Hector D.   01
7/31/57

Elec. Claim Payer ID#
09876599

Company
**ShopMart Stores, Inc.**

Subscriber/Group
00099988765/S45TYU5

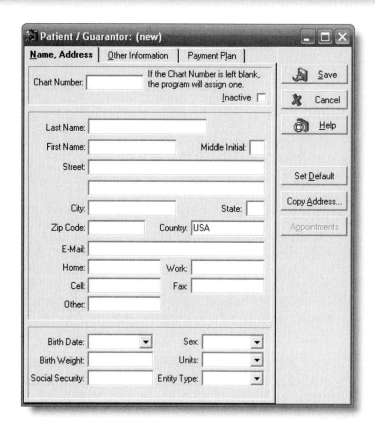

You look at the list of waiting clients and realize that the new patient will not be taken for approximately two hours. It is now around lunch time. Describe how you would suggest that the client take a lunch break and return in 1 and ½ hours. Note: there is a public cafeteria in the building.

_____

_____

_____

_____

_____

# Terms in the Digestive System

## Word Parts in the Digestive System

These are the major word parts used to form words in the digestive system. When you combine these parts with some of the prefixes and suffixes in Units 2 and 3, you will be able to understand medical terms relating to the digestive system.

| | |
|---|---|
| append(o), appendic(o) | appendix |
| bucc(o) | cheek |
| cec(o) | cecum |
| chol(e), cholo- | bile |
| cholangi(o) | bile vessel |
| cholecyst(o) | gallbladder |
| choledoch(o) | common bile duct |
| col(o), colon(o) | colon |
| duoden(o) | duodenum |
| enter(o) | intestines |
| esophag(o) | esophagus |
| gastr(o) | stomach |
| gloss(o) | tongue |
| gluc(o) | glucose |
| glyc(o) | sugar |
| glycogen(o) | glycogen |

| hepat(o) | liver |
| ile(o) | ileum |
| jejun(o) | jejunum |
| labi(o) | lip |
| or(o) | mouth |
| pancreat(o) | pancreas |
| pharyng(o) | pharynx |
| proct(o) | anus, rectum |
| pylor(o) | pylorus |
| rect(o) | rectum |
| sial(o) | saliva, salivary gland |
| sialaden(o) | salivary gland |
| sigmoid(o) | sigmoid colon |
| steat(o) | fats |
| stomat(o) | mouth |

After practicing word building and terminology exercises related to the digestive system, you will learn about searching for a job in a medical facility that specializes in gastrointestinal disorders.

# Exercises in the Digestive System

## Building Terms

For each of the following definitions, provide a term using digestive system word parts as well as prefixes and suffixes you learned in Units 2 and 3.

1. radiographic imaging of the bile ducts: _____

2. fungal infection of the intestines: _____

3. instrument for viewing the colon: _____

4. intestinal hernia: _____

5. destruction of pancreatic tissue: _____

6. of the cheeks and gums: _____.

7. calcification in the appendix: _____

8. rupture of the liver: _____

9. surgical reconstruction of the rectum: _____

10. inflammation of a bile duct: _____

11. surgical formation of a passage from the stomach to the intestines: _____

12. intestinal contraction: _____

13. dilation of the stomach: _____

14. inflammation of the colon: _____

15. poisonous to the liver: _____

16. incision into the cecum: _____

17. gallstone in the bile duct: _____

18. intestinal virus: _____

19. stomach pain: _____

20. inflammation of the rectum: _____

## Completing Terms

Complete the following terms by adding a prefix or suffix to the word or word part given here.

1. surgical puncture of the intestines: entero_____

2. surgical removal of the appendix: append_____

3. surgical opening created in the cecum: ceco_____

4. inflammation of the duodenum: duoden_____

5. downward displacement of the colon: colo_____

6. surgical repair of the esophagus: esophago_____

7. inflammation of the gallbladder: cholecyst_____

8. surgical opening created in the colon: colo_____

9. suturing of the rectum: procto_____

10. surgical fixing of the cecum: ceco_____

11. removal of the gallbladder stone: cholelitho_____

12. surgical removal of the colon: col_____

13. intestinal disease: entero_____

14. enlargement of the liver and spleen: hepatospleno_____

15. rectal hernia: procto_____

## Finding the Word Parts

Break each of the following terms into words or word parts. Give the definition of the term as well as the meaning of each word or word part.

1. hepatocarcinoma: _____

   _____

2. cholecystoduodenostomy: _____

   _____

3. gastroparesis: _____

   _____

4. pylorospasm: _____

   _____

5. proctosigmoidoscopy: _____

   _____

6. oromandibular: _____

   _____

7. sialoadenitis: _____

   _____

8. ileocecal: _____

   _____

9. enterococcus: _____

   _____

**10.** gastroenterocolitis: _____

_____

**11.** esophagogastroduodenoscopy: _____

_____

**12.** gastrojejunostomy: _____

_____

**13.** glycopenia: _____

_____

**14.** jejunoileostomy: _____

_____

**15.** labiodental: _____

_____

## Proofreading and Understanding Terms

Write the correct spelling and definition in the blank to the right of any misspelled words. If the spelling is correct, write C.

**1.** uvola: _____

**2.** gastroentrology: _____

**3.** pilorus: _____

**4.** jejunum: _____

**5.** bilirubin: _____

**6.** dysphogia: _____

**7.** regorgitation: _____

**8.** intussusception: _____

**9.** volvolus: _____

**10.** devirticulitis: _____

**11.** hemorhoids: _____

**12.** incontinence: _____

**13.** asites: _____

**14.** sirrhosis: _____

**15.** jaundice: _____

The following resume for a person seeking a position as a radiologic technician has at least three errors. List the errors.

---

**Marlene Johnson**

45 Taylor Street
Hampton, RI 56565
e-mail: mjtech@yahoo.com
Cell Phone: 565-666-7777

OBJECTIVE:    To find a job in radiology as an immaging technician.

SUMMARY:    As a recent graduate of Trion Career College, I am trained in the use of multiple radiologic modalities. My state certificotion was awarded on July 15.

EDUCATION:    2006–2008: Trion Career College: Certificate in Radiologic Imaging

2006: Hampton High School: Diploma

EXPERIENCE:    2008: Internship at Radiology Associates, Hampton, RI. Duties included patient intake, assisting technician in x-ray and imaging.

2006–2008: Wesley Stores: Cashier; part-time

2004–2006: McDonald's: Clerk; part-time

ACTIVITIES:    Band member in high school; Red Cross Vounteer; member, soccer team (senior year of high school)

REFERENCES:    available un request

---

_____

_____

_____

## Filling in the Blanks

1. Saliva contains _____ that help break down food.

2. The grinding of food by the teeth is known as _____.

3. Food is moved through the digestive system by coordinated muscular contractions called _____.

4. The stomach is divided into _____ regions.

5. The large intestine includes the _____, rectum, and anus.

6. The liver produces _____.

7. Amylase is an enzyme secreted by the _____.

8. Gastric ulcers are usually caused by a(n) _____.

9. Colorectal cancer can be detected early in a(n) _____.

10. Heartburn can be neutralized by the use of a(n) _____.

## True or False

Circle T for true or F for false.

1. Chyme is waste expelled from the body.     T     F

2. The jejunum is part of the large intestine.     T     F

3. The ileum is part of the small intestine.     T     F

4. Anorexia nervosa is an eating disorder in which frequent purging may occur.     T     F

5. GERD is a disease of the small intestines.     T     F

6. Polyps in the intestines are always cancerous.     T     F

7. Colic frequently becomes a lifelong problem.     T     F

8. Hepatitis A is a chronic infection of the liver.     T     F

9. A barium enema is used in an upper GI series.     T     F

10. Loss of the appendix can be fatal.     T     F

## Using a Dictionary

In your allied health dictionary, go to the entry gastr(o) and find eight words that describe stomach ailments and/or surgical procedures. Break each word into parts and define the word.

1. _____

_____

2. _____

_____

3. _____

_____

4. _____

_____

5. _____

_____

6. _____

_____

7. _____

_____

8. _____

_____

Name _____

Class _____ Date _____

## Writing the Medical Term

For each of the following descriptions, write the proper medical term or an alternative medical term.

1. spit: _____

2. stomach ache: _____

3. intestinal infection: _____

4. lower jaw bone: _____

5. bowel movement: _____

6. swallowing food: _____

7. gas: _____

8. removal of one or more lobes of the liver: _____

9. examination of the colon: _____

10. agent that neutralizes stomach acid: _____

## Crossword

## CLUES

### Across

1. Condition with tongue attached incorrectly

6. Raised area on tongue

10. Projection from soft palate

11. Of the liver

12. Place at which feces exits body

14. Bottom part of small intestine

17. _____ intestine

18. Pouch at the top of the large intestine

20. Pharynx

22. _____ intestine

23. Fleshy part of mouth that moves

26. Semisolid mass in stomach

27. Agent that relieves constipation

29. Inflammation of the bile ducts

31. Eating disorder

32. Laxative

33. Connects pharynx to stomach

### Down

2. Sick feeling

3. Organ that secretes bile

4. Fat in the blood

5. Inflammation of the ileum

7. Agent that prevents emesis

8. Pancreatic enzyme

9. _____ canal

13. Place where food is broken down

15. Inflammation of the intestines

16. Belching

18. Removal of gallbladder

19. Membrane that attaches intestines to the abdominal wall

21. Appendage

24. Twisted intestinal blockage

25. Appendix

26. Combining form for the common bile duct

28. Secreted by liver

30. _____ palate

## Finding a Job

You are a graduate of a program in medical assisting. For two years, you have worked in the practice of a gastroenterologist. You and your family are moving to another state in two months. You have given notice to your boss and have gotten a great recommendation. You are planning to spend the next two months searching for a job in the new location and will take a few days off to go to interviews if you can schedule them.

## Making up a Resume

In Unit 1, you saw sample resumes. Using the form below, make up a resume for someone who has graduated from a two-year medical assisting program, has worked for a gastroenterologist for two years, and is planning to move to another state where he or she is seeking a similar job.

OBJECTIVE: _____

_____

SUMMARY: _____

_____

_____

_____

EDUCATION: _____

_____

_____

EXPERIENCE: _____

_____

_____

_____

_____

ACTIVITIES: _____

_____

REFERENCES: _____

_____

## Searching on the Internet

Go to several job search sites such as Monster.com and Careerbuilder.com and online newspaper sites in another state. Find at least three appropriate jobs for the person for whom you created a resume above. Briefly list the ads here.

1. _____

   _____

2. _____

   _____

3. _____

   _____

## Applying on the Internet

Write a cover letter that could be used for each of the jobs.

_____

_____

_____

_____

_____

_____

_____

_____

_____

## Interviewing

You are able to schedule two interviews. Write a brief paragraph describing several questions you might have for the interviewer.

_____

_____

_____

_____

_____

_____

# Terms in the Endocrine System

## Word Parts in the Endocrine System

These are the major word parts used to form words in the endocrine system. When you combine these parts with some of the prefixes and suffixes in Units 2 and 3, you will be able to understand medical terms relating to the endocrine system.

| | |
|---|---|
| aden(o) | gland |
| adren(o), adrenal(o) | adrenal glands |
| gluc(o) | glucose |
| glyc(o) | glycogen |
| pancreat(o) | pancreas |
| parathyroid(o) | parathyroid gland |
| thyr(o), thyroid(o) | thyroid gland |

After practicing word building and terminology exercises related to the endocrine system, you will learn about working in a hospital.

## Exercises in the Endocrine System

### Building Terms

For each of the following definitions, provide a term using endocrine system word parts as well as prefixes and suffixes you learned in Units 2 and 3.

1. destruction of pancreatic tissue: _____

2. tumor derived from glandular tissue: _____

3. glucose formation: _____

4. adrenal inflammation: _____

5. sugar deficiency in an organ: _____

6. increase in adrenal gland size: _____

7. presence of sugar in the blood: _____

8. involving the adrenal cortex: _____

9. surgical incision into the pancreas: _____

10. thyroid inflammation: _____

## Completing Terms

Complete the following terms by adding a prefix or suffix to the word or word part given here.

1. abnormal glandular condition: aden_____

2. inflammation of the pancreas: pancreat_____

3. glycogen formation: glyco_____

4. removal of an adrenal gland: adrenal_____

5. removal of the thyroid: thyroid_____

6. glandular inflammation: aden_____

7. removal of the parathyroid: parathyoid_____

8. adrenal disease: adreno_____

9. oversecretion of thyroid: _____thyroidism.

10. undersecrtion of thyroid: _____thyroidism.

## Finding the Word Parts

Break each of the following terms into words or word parts. Give the definition of the term as well as the meaning of each word or word part.

1. glycolysis: _____

_____

2. homeostasis: _____

_____

3. thyromegaly: _____

_____

Name _____

Class _____ Date _____

___

4. hyperparathyroidism: _____

_____

5. adrenocorticohyperplasia: _____

_____

6. thyrotoxicosis: _____

_____

7. polydipsia: _____

_____

8. hyperglycemia: _____

_____

9. hyperinsulinism: _____

_____

10. thyroglobulin: _____

_____

## Proofreading and Understanding Terms

Write the correct spelling and definition in the blank to the right of any misspelled words. If the spelling is correct, write C.

1. pinal gland: _____     6. triiodothyronine: _____

2. diabetes melitis: _____     7. norepineprine: _____

3. retinapathy: _____     8. glicosuria: _____

4. hipopituitarism: _____     9. hypothalamus: _____

5. melotonin: _____     10. adrenocoticotropic: _____

As a learning exercise you were asked to list the major endocrine glands and their functions. Here is your list. Proofread it and list any corrections below.

| hypothalomus | stimulate or inhibit pituitary secretions |
|---|---|
| neurohypopysis | increase water reabsorption<br>stimulates uterine contractions and lactition<br>stimulates production of melinin |
| adenohypopysis | stimulate bone and muscle growth<br>stimulates thyroid gland to secrete hormones<br>stimulates secretion of adrenal cortex hormones |
| thyroid | regulates metabolism; stimulates growth |
| parathyroid | increase blood calcium as necessary to maintain homeotasis |
| adrenal medolla<br><br><br>adrenal cortex | work with the sympathetic nervous system to react to stress<br><br>affect metabolism, growth, and aid inelectrolyte and fluid balances |
| pancreas | maintain homeosasis in blood glucose concentration |
| ovaries | promote development of female sex characteristics, menstrual cycle, reproductive functions |
| testes | promote development of male sex characteristics, sperm production |

_____

_____

_____

_____

_____

_____

_____

## Filling In the Blanks

1. Glands that release hormones directly into the blood are _____ glands.

2. The hypophysis is also known as the _____ gland.

3. Glands that release hormones through ducts are _____ glands.

4. Calcium in the blood is regulated by hormones from the _____ glands.

5. Glands release substances known as _____.

6. The islets of Langerhans are located in the _____.

7. Growth hormone is secreted by the _____ gland.

8. Blood sugar is lowered by _____.

9. Polyuria is often a symptom of _____.

10. Hypersecretion of growth hormone during childhood can cause _____.

## True or False

Circle T for true or F for false.

1. The thymus is known as the body's master gland.     T     F

2. Pigment in the skin is produced by the substance melanin.     T     F

3. Insulin is secreted by the parathyroid glands.     T     F

4. The adrenal glands are located right on top of to the kidneys.     T     F

5. Epinephrine lowers the heart rate.     T     F

6. Type II diabetes is a type of autoimmune disease.     T     F

7. Melatonin helps regulate the sleep cycle.     T     F

8. Testosterone is the most abundant male hormone.     T     F

9. A goiter is a swelling of the thyroid gland.     T     F

10. Graves' disease is caused by hypothyroidism.     T     F

## Using a Dictionary

Using your allied health dictionary, describe the following endocrine tests.

1. GTT: _____

_____

**2.** FBS: _____

_____

**3.** TFT: _____

_____

## Word Find

In the following puzzle, draw a line around at least 20 words pertaining to the integumentary system. The words can be horizontal, vertical, diagonal, or upside-down. Write the words on the rules provided. If you do not know the meaning of a word, look it up in your allied health dictionary and make a flash card for future review.

| r | b | k | a | m | s | i | l | i | r | i | v | g | w | q | c | e | t | u | o |
|---|---|---|---|---|---|---|---|---|---|---|---|---|---|---|---|---|---|---|---|
| p | s | a | n | j | l | u | o | p | e | a | n | l | t | h | o | t | o | u | p |
| l | a | n | d | g | e | h | i | k | o | p | l | u | c | y | e | y | a | a | v |
| h | a | c | r | o | m | e | g | a | l | y | j | c | o | p | p | l | c | i | n |
| e | y | k | o | o | p | l | l | g | e | l | y | o | v | h | y | o | m | m | a |
| r | y | n | g | a | w | j | y | r | i | k | n | s | e | o | x | r | w | e | y |
| s | n | q | e | z | h | y | c | a | m | k | t | u | w | p | h | t | i | c | k |
| e | d | d | n | a | l | g | o | v | k | o | p | r | b | h | q | c | n | y | i |
| t | s | y | f | j | k | l | g | e | w | e | q | i | b | y | n | e | m | l | j |
| e | s | w | r | a | z | w | e | s | h | i | l | a | d | s | h | l | h | g | w |
| b | i | w | q | a | h | l | n | d | o | w | i | p | j | i | a | e | n | o | m |
| a | q | i | e | k | v | l | v | i | r | z | n | i | p | s | w | o | k | p | g |
| i | c | o | t | k | s | o | l | s | m | s | i | f | r | a | w | d | z | y | e |
| d | l | i | g | h | s | j | l | e | o | y | e | w | c | n | s | k | l | h | u |
| a | z | n | d | y | y | a | n | a | n | t | i | k | c | t | y | m | w | m | i |
| o | k | s | i | o | b | m | q | s | e | x | o | c | r | i | n | e | a | l | i |
| c | s | u | h | w | s | x | u | e | m | k | u | p | w | b | t | v | s | d | n |
| t | l | l | m | l | o | i | w | s | c | p | a | n | c | r | e | a | s | q | a |
| n | l | i | w | t | y | p | s | o | s | i | s | j | k | l | a | n | e | w | x |
| u | e | n | l | o | y | p | g | l | x | u | m | s | i | t | n | a | g | i | g |
| j | c | k | u | n | r | q | l | u | m | n | m | c | y | u | k | o | p | l | f |
| a | a | b | a | n | m | e | e | h | a | i | r | u | s | o | c | y | l | g | x |
| i | t | t | l | b | c | c | t | w | s | v | g | n | j | k | b | d | y | w | z |
| n | e | m | i | a | l | s | l | i | c | x | e | q | d | i | o | r | e | t | s |
| t | b | m | h | l | i | n | i | n | o | t | i | c | l | a | c | w | y | o | p |
| z | h | p | u | l | p | h | q | b | m | g | k | a | w | k | l | m | i | u | f |
| t | l | b | x | b | m | k | g | t | d | a | d | r | e | n | a | l | i | n | e |
| a | w | d | u | c | t | l | e | s | s | g | l | a | n | d | d | g | j | m | f |

a. _____    n. _____

b. _____    o. _____

c. _____    p. _____

d. _____    q. _____

e. _____    r. _____

f. _____    s. _____

g. _____    t. _____

h. _____    u. _____

i. _____    v. _____

j. _____    w. _____

k. _____    x. _____

l. _____    y. _____

m. _____    z. _____

## Working in a Hospital

You are a hospital billing clerk at a major city hospital. The hospital serves many people on Medicare and Medicaid. Privacy concerns are a fundamental element of how you handle information as are patient rights. Read the following summary of patient rights under HIPAA rules and the patient's bill of rights. Write a paragraph explaining how it affects your job.

---

### HIPAA Rules

- Your healthcare provider and your insurance company must give you a privacy policy explaining how they'll use and disclose health information.
- You can ask for copies of all information, and make appropriate changes to it. You can also ask for a history of any disclosures.
- If someone wants to share your health information, you have to give your formal consent.
- You have the right to complain to the government about violations of HIPAA rules.
- Health information is to be used only for health purposes. Without your consent, it can't be used to help banks decide whether to give you credit, or by potential employers to decide whether to give you a job.
- When your health information gets shared, only the minimum necessary amount of information should be disclosed.
- Mental health records get an extra level of protection.

## Patients' Bill of Rights

- The right to considerate and respectful care.
- The right to relevant, current, and understandable information about their diagnosis, treatment, and prognosis.
- The right to make decisions about the planned care and the right to refuse care.
- The right to have an advance directive (such as a living will) concerning treatment if they become incapacitated.
- The right to privacy in all procedures, examinations, and discussions of treatment.
- The right to confidential handling of all information and records about their care.
- The right to look over and have all records about their care explained.
- The right to suggest changes in the planned care or to transfer to another facility.
- The right to be informed about the business relationships among the hospital and other facilities that are part of the treatment and care.
- The right to decide whether to take part in experimental treatments.
- The right to understand their care options after a hospital stay.
- The right to know about the hospital's policies for settling disputes and to examine and receive an explanation of all charges.

_____

_____

_____

_____

_____

_____

_____

_____

UNIT **16**

# Terms in the Sensory System

## Word Parts in the Sensory System

These are the major word parts used to form words in the sensory system. When you combine these parts with some of the prefixes and suffixes in Units 2 and 3, you will be able to understand medical terms relating to the sensory system.

| | |
|---|---|
| audi(o), audit(o) | hearing |
| blephar(o) | eyelid |
| cochle(o) | cochlea |
| cor(o), core(o) | pupil |
| corne(o) | cornea |
| cycl(o) | ciliary body |
| dacry(o) | tears |
| ir(o), irid(o) | iris |
| kerat(o) | cornea |
| mastoid(o) | mastoid process |
| myring(o) | eardrum, middle ear |
| nas(o) | nose |
| ocul(o) | eye |
| ophthalm(o) | eye |
| opt(o), optic(o) | eye |
| phac(o), phak(o) | lens |
| pupill(o) | pupil |
| retin(o) | retina |
| scler(o) | white of the eye |
| scot(o) | darkness |
| tympan(o) | eardrum, middle ear |
| uve(o) | uvea |

After practicing word building and terminology exercises related to the sensory system, you will learn about working for an optical center.

# Exercises in the Sensory System

## Building Terms

For each of the following definitions, provide a term using sensory system word parts as well as prefixes and suffixes you learned in Units 2 and 3.

1. discharge of tears with blood: _____

2. surgical repair of the tympanic membrane: _____

3. softening of the lens of an eye: _____

4. drooping of the eyelid: _____

5. instrument for measuring the cornea: _____

6. pain in the iris: _____

7. surgical repair of the eardrum: _____

8. bulging of the sclera: _____

9. involving the nose and tear ducts: _____

10. of the cornea and sclera: _____

11. paralysis of the ciliary muscle: _____

12. splitting of the retina into layers: _____

13. inflammation of the mastoid process: _____

14. swelling of the eyelid: _____

15. instrument for measuring sound: _____

16. calculus in the tear duct: _____

17. fungal infection of the cornea: _____

18. medical specialty that treats the eyes: _____

19. specialist who prescribes corrective lenses: _____

20. inflammation of the uvea: _____

## Completing Terms

Complete the following terms by adding a prefix or suffix to the word or word part given here.

1. inflammation of the tear gland: dacryoaden_____

2. eye pain: oculo_____

3. softening of the iris: irido_____

4. instrument for measuring eye function: ophthalmo_____

5. device for measuring hearing: audio_____

6. incision into the mastoid process: mastoido_____

7. device for observing the pupil: pupillo_____

8. inflammation of the nasopharynx: nasopharyng_____

9. drooping of the iris: irido_____

10. incision into the eyelid: blepharo_____

11. discharge of tears containing pus: dacryopyo_____

12. inflammation of the iris and ciliary body: iridocycl_____

13. surgical removal of the eardrum: myring_____

14. softening or thinning of the sclera: sclero_____

15. inflammation of the retina: retin_____

## Finding the Word Parts

Break each of the following terms into words or word parts. Give the definition of the term as well as the meaning of each word or word part.

1. blepharophimosis: _____

_____

2. uveoscleritis: _____

_____

3. corectopia: _____

_____

4. phacoemulsification: _____

_____

5. dacryocystorhinostomy: _____

_____

6. iridorrhexis: _____

_____

7. cochleovestibular: _____

_____

8. ossiculectomy: _____

_____

9. coreoplasty: _____

_____

10. myringomycosis: _____

_____

## Proofreading and Understanding Terms

Write the correct spelling and definition in the blank to the right of any misspelled words. If the spelling is correct, write C.

1. otorinolaringology: _____

2. coclea: _____

3. decibel: _____

4. eustachian: _____

5. temparomandiblar: _____

6. tinitus: _____

7. lingal: _____

8. ossicals: _____

9. timpanum: _____

10. Menier's disease: _____

A customer needs a hearing aid. You have been instructed to give her a statement of the treatment and the costs for her to read since you will not be able to discuss it with her easily. Proofread the statement and list any errors you find.

---

Dear Mrs. Jones,

Doctor Alvarez asked me to give you this statement of treatment and costs for you in-ear hearing aid. You will need a total of 4 visits at the beginning.

The first visit will be a compehensive evoluation of your hearing difficulties. It will take about two hours. You should bring a firend or family member along to this appointment.

The second visit will be a fitting that will be followed by two subsequint appoinmtets for adjustments.

The total cost including the evaluation and fittings is $795.00. As a Medicare recipient, you will be covered for 80 percent of this or $525.00. The remainder can be paid in partial payments arranged with this office over a period of four months.

Please let me know if you understand this by signing below.

---

_____

_____

_____

_____

## Filling In the Blanks

1. The aqueous humor is produced by the _____ body.

2. Cloudy vision is usually caused by a _____.

3. The malleus, stapes, and incus are known as the _____.

4. In the retina, _____ are sensitive to light.

5. Color is sensed by _____ in the retina.

6. Earwax is also known as _____.

7. The colored area of the eye is the _____.

8. Light rays enter the eye through the _____.

9. Double vision is also called _____.

10. Hearing loss as a result of old age is _____.

## True or False

Circle T for true or F for false.

1. The auricle is part of the inner ear.     T     F

2. Blepharitis is an inflammation of the middle ear.     T     F

3. Otitis medica is a common childhood ear infection.     T     F

4. A postnasal drip is usually infectious.     T     F

5. An audiologist measures the eyes for lenses.     T     F

6. Anosmia is the loss of the sense of smell.     T     F

7. Tinnitus is an infectious disease.     T     F

8. Otalgia occurs in the eyes.     T     F

9. Retinitis occurs in the ears.     T     F

10. A mydriatic contracts the pupils.     T     F

## Using a Dictionary

Using your allied health dictionary, look up each of the five senses. Describe the location and major organs of each of the senses.

1. _____

_____

_____

_____

_____

2. _____

_____

_____

_____

_____

3. _____

_____

_____

_____

_____

4. _____

_____

_____

_____

_____

5. _____

_____

_____

_____

_____

## Writing the Medical Term

For each of the following descriptions, write the proper medical term or an alternative medical term.

**1.** runny nose: _____

**2.** crying: _____

**3.** loss of the sense of smell: _____

**4.** dizziness: _____

**5.** eardrum: _____

**6.** pinkeye: _____

**7.** sty: _____

**8.** crosseye: _____

**9.** nearsightedness: _____

**10.** farsightedness: _____

## Word Find

In the following puzzle, draw a line around at least 20 words pertaining to the integumentary system. The words can be horizontal, vertical, diagonal, or upside-down. Write the words on the rules provided. If you do not know the meaning of a word, look it up in your allied health dictionary and make a flash card for future review.

| a | u | n | n | x | i | a | i | p | o | l | a | t | c | y | n | s | e | n | d |
|---|---|---|---|---|---|---|---|---|---|---|---|---|---|---|---|---|---|---|---|
| k | i | s | o | n | a | h | e | a | r | w | m | k | z | a | j | k | m | e | l |
| q | x | s | a | g | h | t | h | r | u | j | k | l | o | n | k | d | c | n | m |
| e | y | e | b | r | o | w | e | x | i | g | a | c | a | i | w | i | j | m | k |
| m | l | n | t | s | g | t | w | q | n | u | j | t | h | t | b | p | j | i | k |
| t | v | f | b | e | p | w | q | n | r | j | k | i | y | e | a | l | y | o | p |
| o | v | a | b | o | q | r | t | i | y | k | l | p | l | r | b | o | m | t | x |
| u | q | e | i | a | g | h | c | i | l | i | a | r | y | w | j | p | l | i | u |
| c | e | d | w | j | i | l | j | m | l | s | w | b | n | x | r | i | y | c | a |
| h | s | h | j | k | e | w | q | m | c | o | p | l | j | i | d | a | s | e | i |
| n | s | n | e | l | j | l | z | a | a | i | p | o | y | m | r | w | h | m | p |
| i | o | k | l | p | a | x | a | t | t | h | k | i | l | c | k | i | o | l | o |
| b | n | y | e | e | m | k | c | h | a | l | a | z | i | o | n | k | t | l | r |
| w | g | i | n | c | u | s | n | j | r | t | q | v | m | n | u | o | i | i | t |
| s | f | r | y | c | v | z | t | e | a | r | s | j | k | e | o | t | p | n | s |
| z | o | b | w | x | e | j | k | l | c | i | o | a | x | s | w | o | q | t | e |
| c | l | r | y | m | a | b | c | t | t | m | w | j | k | l | a | l | v | a | w |
| m | j | u | k | o | p | i | l | l | a | k | a | n | o | e | g | o | v | s | a |
| a | l | e | j | h | a | r | i | i | i | s | b | r | a | j | l | g | u | t | l |
| x | v | t | w | q | n | k | l | o | n | p | x | w | g | q | a | i | m | e | l |
| e | t | s | u | e | l | l | a | m | h | d | a | m | z | o | q | s | t | h | k |
| a | y | l | a | n | t | y | c | s | a | e | n | t | r | a | i | t | u | n | a |
| r | z | x | t | y | u | m | k | i | l | l | a | e | c | b | e | d | q | l | i |
| d | d | g | n | i | r | a | e | h | k | l | v | r | s | s | r | t | u | y | n |
| r | h | j | v | c | e | t | c | j | k | l | u | i | d | s | s | c | a | a | a |
| u | x | v | b | n | m | o | p | t | i | c | i | a | n | w | a | q | u | i | o |
| m | g | a | n | a | c | u | s | i | s | x | u | l | i | m | o | p | l | b | e |
| p | i | n | k | e | y | e | m | k | n | i | a | r | t | s | e | y | e | w | t |

a. _____     n. _____

b. _____     o. _____

c. _____     p. _____

d. _____     q. _____

e. _____     r. _____

f. _____     s. _____

g. _____     t. _____

h. _____     u. _____

i. _____     v. _____

j. _____     w. _____

k. _____     x. _____

l. _____     y. _____

m. _____     z. _____

# Working in an Optical Center

You are an assistant in an optical center where there is one optometrist giving examinations and prescribing lenses. The center also sells eyeglasses and contact lenses. Your job is to greet the clients, explain the process and show the available frames and shades of lenses. For clients getting their eye examination at the center, you fit walk-ins into the schedule if possible and you schedule appointments for people who call or stop by. For clients who bring in an ophthalmologist's prescription, you work with them to choose frames.

It is a particularly busy Saturday morning. There are three scheduled eye examinations that take about 30 minutes each. There are four walk-ins looking for examinations and there are five people who just need to choose frames. You and a coworker have to handle all the clients. You have people sign in.

For the scheduled appointments, you have folders ready from previous examinations. The first client has no change in her prescription and the optometrist asks you to show her a selection of frames. You note that she needs bifocals and will require a slightly larger frame. She would like to buy the tiny half frames that will not work. Write a paragraph describing how you would tell her what she needs and try to guide her toward the right style without offending her.

_____

_____

_____

_____

_____

_____

She chooses frames which cost $95.00. The bifocals will cost an additional $125.00. There is no tax on eyeglasses in your state. You write up a bill and ask for a 30 percent deposit. Fill in the missing information on the bill below.

Cost of lenses: _____

Cost of frames: _____

Total: _____

Less deposit of 30% _____ paid on _____.

Total due when picking up eyeglasses: _____

You make sure she signs the receipt and you mark her folder paid in full. You give her a card for the next week showing her what hours you are open for her to pick up her glasses.

# Terms in Pharmacology

## Word Parts in Pharmacology

These are the major word parts used to form words in pharmacology. When you combine these parts with some of the prefixes and suffixes in Units 2 and 3, you will be able to understand medical terms relating to pharmacology.

| | |
|---|---|
| chem(o) | chemical |
| pharmac(o) | drugs |
| pyr(o) | fever |
| tox(o), toxi, toxico | poison |

## Abbreviations in Pharmacology

In the field of pharmacology, many abbreviations are used in writing orders and filling prescriptions. Some abbreviations (especially when handwritten) can cause confusion and lead to medical errors, sometimes fatal ones. Refer to Appendix B starting on page 220 to learn more about how to avoid such errors. Listed below are abbreviations commonly used in pharmacology.

### Abbreviation Meaning

| | |
|---|---|
| aa, aa | of each |
| a.c. | before meals (Latin *ante cibum*), usually one-half hour preceding a meal |
| ad | up to |
| a.d., AD | right ear (Latin *auris dexter*) |
| ad lib | freely (Latin *ad libitum*), as often as desired |
| AM, a.m., A | morning (Latin *ante meridiem*) |

| a.s., AS | left ear (Latin *auris sinister*) |
| a.u., AU | each ear (Latin *auris uterque*) |
| BID, b.i.d. | twice a day (Latin *bis in die*) |
| c, c | with |
| cap., caps. | capsule |
| cc., cc | cubic centimeter |
| comp. | compound |
| cx | contraindicated |
| DAW | dispense as written |
| dil. | dilute |
| disc, DC, dc | discontinue |
| disp. | dispense |
| div. | divide |
| DW | distilled water |
| $D_5W$ | dextrose 5% in water |
| dx, Dx | diagnosis |
| elix. | elixir |
| e.m.p. | as directed (Latin *ex modo praescripto*) |
| ex aq. | in water |
| ext. | extract |
| FDA | Food and Drug Administration |
| fld. ext. | fluid extract |
| FUO | fever of unknown origin |
| g, gm | gram |
| gr | grain, gram |
| gtt | drop |
| H | hypodermic |
| h. | every hour (Latin *hora*) |

| h.s. | at bedtime (Latin *hora somni* [hour of sleep]) |
| IM | intramuscular |
| inj | injection |
| IV | intravenous |
| mcg | microgram |
| mEq | milliequivalent |
| mg | milligram |
| ml | milliliter |
| n., noct. | night (Latin *nocte*) |
| non rep. | do not repeat |
| NPO | nothing by mouth |
| NPO p MN | nothing by mouth after midnight |
| N.S., NS | normal saline |
| NSAID | nonsteroidal anti-inflammatory drug |
| N&V | nausea and vomiting |
| o.d. | right eye (Latin *oculus dexter*) |
| oint., ung. | ointment, unguent |
| o.l. | left eye |
| o.s. | left eye (Latin *oculus sinister*) |
| OTC | over the counter |
| o.u. | each eye |
| oz. | ounce |
| p | post, after |
| p.c. | after meals (Latin *post cibum*), one-half hour after a meal |
| PDR | *Physician's Desk Reference* |
| PM, p.m., P | afternoon (Latin *post meridiem*) |

| p.o. | by mouth (Latin *per os*) |
| PRN, p.r.n. | repeat as needed (Latin *pro re nata*) |
| pulv., pwdr | powder |
| qam | every morning |
| q.d. | every day (Latin *quaque dies*) |
| q.h. | every hour |
| q.i.d. | four times a day |
| QNS | quantity not sufficient |
| q.o.d. | every other day |
| q.s. | sufficient quantity |
| R | rectal |
| Rx | prescription |
| s, s̄ | without |
| Sig. | patient directions such as route and timing of medication (Latin *signa*, inscription) |
| SL | sublingual |
| sol., soln. | solution |
| s.o.s. | if there is need |
| sp. | spirit |
| ss, s̄s̄ | one-half |
| stat | immediately |
| subc, subq, s.c. | subcutaneously |
| supp., suppos | suppository |
| susp. | suspension |
| sym, Sym, Sx | symptom |
| syr. | syrup |
| tab. | tablet |
| tbsp. | tablespoonful |
| t.i.d. | three times a day |
| tinct., tr. | tincture |

| TPN | total parenteral nutrition |
|-----|---------------------------|
| TPR | temperature, pulse, respirations |
| tsp. | teaspoonful |
| U, u | unit |
| u.d. | as directed |
| ung. | ointment |
| U.S.P. | *United States Pharmacopeia* |

# Exercises in Pharmacology

## Building Terms

For each of the following definitions, provide a term using pharmacology word parts as well as prefixes and suffixes you learned in Units 2 and 3.

1. study of drugs: _____

2. study of poisonous substances: _____

3. treatment of disease using chemicals: _____

4. producing toxic substances: _____

5. causing a fever: _____

## Matching

Write the letter of the meaning of the abbreviation in the space provided.

1. NPO _____

2. t.i.d. _____

3. p.c. _____

4. stat _____

5. TPN _____

6. c _____

7. dil _____

8. dx _____

a. total parenteral nurtrition

b. with

c. dilute

d. each ear

e. after meals

f. milligrams

g. suspension

h. hypodermic

9. ex aq. _____

10. a.u. _____

11. IM _____

12. ml _____

13. mg _____

14. H _____

15. q.h. _____

16. a.s. _____

17. u _____

18. tsp. _____

19. susp. _____

20. a.c. _____

i. intramuscularly

j. milliter

k. teaspoon

l. in water

m. diagnosis

n. three times a day

o. before meals

p. unit

q. left ear

r. immediately

s. nothing by mouth

t. every hour

## True or False

Circle T for true or F for false.

1. All drugs require a prescription.     T     F

2. Intramuscular and intradermal administration are the same thing.     T     F

3. Subcutaneously means beneath the skin.     T     F

4. An infusion is inhaled through the nose.     T     F

5. Hormones are both natural and synthetic.     T     F

6. Generic drugs are usually less expensive.     T     F

7. An antidote relieves edema.     T     F

8. Sublingually is under the tongue.     T     F

9. A suppository is injected into the skin.     T     F

10. A mydriatic contracts the pupils.     T     F

Name _____

Class _____ Date _____

## Using a Dictionary

Using your allied health dictionary, look up at the appendix of abbreviations. Choose five abbreviations and describe the meaning of each.

1. _____
   _____
   _____
   _____
   _____

2. _____
   _____
   _____
   _____
   _____

3. _____
   _____
   _____
   _____
   _____

4. _____
   _____
   _____
   _____
   _____

**5.** _____

_____

_____

_____

_____

## Working in a Pharmacy

You are a pharmacy technician at a large retail store. One of your major tasks is to provide customer service. Many of the customers are elderly and use the Medicare prescription plan which they find confusing. You use a computer to calculate cost. Customers are sometimes shocked at what they have to pay for copayments. Describe the ways in which you might handle a tense situation in which a customer claims you are overcharging him.

_____

_____

_____

_____

The Internet can be useful to you for learning about medications both as a pharmacy tech student and as a consumer. Go to www.fda.gov, click on drugs and then click on drugs@FDA. Choose any 10 drugs at random and write down whether they are prescription or not, the company that manufactures them, and in how many different dosages they are available.

_____

_____

_____

_____

_____

_____

_____

_____

# Medical Terminology Review

The review in this unit covers the previous 17 units as well as a short review of complementary and alternative medicine (CAM). If you have not yet studied CAM, please review Appendix D, "Complementary and Alternative Medicine," before completing the exercises in the CAM section. For the other units, you will find the following three appendices very helpful.

1. Appendix A: Combining Forms, Prefixes, and Suffixes
2. Appendix B: Medical Errors and Abbreviations
3. Appendix C Laboratory Testing and Normal Reference Values

## Exercises in Medical Terminology

### Combining Forms, Prefixes, and Suffixes

The following matching exercises test your knowledge of word parts used in medical terminology word building. For any terms you miss, make a flash card for later review. Write the letter of the answer in the space provided.

*Match each word part with its closest definition.*

a. aden(o)

b. blephar(o)

c. nas(o)

d. dermat(o)

e. sperm(o)

f. vas(o)

g. hemi-

h. vesic(o)

1. eyelid____

2. sperm____

3. bladder____

4. blood vessel____

5. gland____

6. nose____

7. half____

8. skin____

*Match each word part with its closest definition*

**a.** cec(o)

**b.** schiz(o)

**c.** cochle(o)

**d.** cholecyst(o)

**e.** maxill(o)

**f.** lacrim(o)

**g.** ped(i)

**h.** pancreat(o)

**9.** cochlea____

**10.** tears____

**11.** pancreas____

**12.** cecum____

**13.** gallbladder____

**14.** split____

**15.** upper jaw____

**16.** foot____

*Match each word part with its closest definition*

**a.** adren(o)

**b.** duoden(o)

**c.** gastr(o)

**d.** tympan(o)

**e.** gonad(o)

**f.** ocul(o)

**g.** append(o)

**h.** cerumin(o)

**17.** eye____

**18.** stomach____

**19.** duodenum____

**20.** eardrum____

**21.** adrenal glands____

**22.** wax____

**23.** sex glands____

**24.** appendix____

*Match each word part with its closest definition*

**a.** col(o)

**b.** thorac(o)

**c.** hepat(o)

**d.** thyroid(o)

**e.** athero

**f.** gingiv(o)

**g.** esophag(o)

**h.** -derma

**25.** esophagus____

**26.** colon____

**27.** thyroid____

**28.** gums____

**29.** liver____

**30.** skin____

**31.** thorax____

**32.** fatty matter____

*Match each word part with its closest definition*

**a.** vertebr(o)

**b.** carcin(o)

**c.** carp(o)

**d.** syring(o)

**e.** neur(o)

**f.** proct(o)

**g.** leuk(o)

**h.** nucle(o)

**33.** white____

**34.** cancer____

**35.** nerve____

**36.** tube____

**37.** wrist____

**38.** vertebra____

**39.** nucleus____

**40.** anus____

*Match each word part with its closest definition*

**a.** mamm(o)

**b.** scapul(o)

**c.** ambi-

**d.** metacarp(o)

**e.** geront(o)

**f.** retin(o)

**g.** chrom(o)

**h.** hydr(o)

**41.** both____

**42.** old age____

**43.** breast____

**44.** color____

**45.** retina____

**46.** water____

**47.** metacarpal____

**48.** scapula____

*Match each word part with its closest definition*

**a.** phag(o)

**b.** stern(o)

**c.** labi(o)

**d.** cervic(o)

**e.** melan(o)

**f.** galact(o)

**g.** gloss(o)

**h.** brachy-

**49.** milk____

**50.** lip____

**51.** sternum____

**52.** black____

**53.** devouring____

**54.** tongue____

**55.** short____

**56.** cervix____

*Match each word part with its closest definition*

**a.** kinesi(o)

**b.** peri-

**c.** ossicul(o)

**d.** -clasis

**e.** exo-

**f.** narco

**g.** thrombo

**h.** crypt(o)

**57.** breaking____

**58.** around____

**59.** blood clot____

**60.** ossicle____

**61.** hidden____

**62.** sleep____

**63.** motion____

**64.** external____

*Match each word part with its closest definition*

**a.** pharyng(o)

**b.** fungi

**c.** jejun(o)

**d.** -graphy

**e.** brady-

**f.** condyl(o)

**g.** inguin(o)

**h.** ankyl(o)

**65.** process of recording____

**66.** fungus____

**67.** knuckle____

**68.** bent____

**69.** pharynx____

**70.** jejunum____

**71.** groin____

**72.** slow____

*Match each word part with its closest definition*

**a.** kyph(o)

**b.** olig(o)-

**c.** ichthy(o)

**d.** -ism

**e.** -ectomy

**f.** rachi(o)

**g.** ovari(o)

**h.** cyst(o)

73. few____

74. removal of____

75. condition____

76. ovary____

77. bladder____

78. spine____

79. hump____

80. scaly____

*Match each word part with its closest definition*

**a.** poly-

**b.** chlor(o)

**c.** bucc(o)

**d.** trache(o)

**e.** immun(o)

**f.** -globin

**g.** apo-

**h.** infra-

81. immunity____

82. cheek____

83. trachea____

84. beneath____

85. many____

86. chlorine__

87. derived____

88. protein____

*Match each word part with its closest definition*

**a.** ischi(o)

**b.** lapar(o)

**c.** hypn(o)

**d.** chondr(o)

**e.** -itis

**f.** bronchiol(o)

**g.** calci(o)

**h.** thalam(o)

**89.** inflammation____

**90.** abdominal wall____

**91.** cartilage____

**92.** thalamus____

**93.** bronchiole____

**94.** sleep____

**95.** calcium____

**96.** ischium____

## Multiple Choice

Write the letter of the correct answer in the space provided. These questions test your general knowledge of medical terminology.

**1.** The system that controls excretion of waste is the _____.

    **a.** sensory system

    **b.** blood system

    **c.** digestive system

    **d.** urinary system

**2.** A gastroscopy is a procedure for examining the _____.

    **a.** liver

    **b.** pancreas

    **c.** gallbladder

    **d.** none of the above

**3.** The blood type that has no antigens is _____.

    **a.** A

    **b.** B

    **c.** O

    **d.** D

4. A vasectomy is performed for _____.

    **a.** cancer control

    **b.** birth control

    **c.** correction of sexual dysfunction

    **d.** increased hormone production

5. Prostate cancer usually occurs because of exposure to _____.

    **a.** tobacco

    **b.** asbestos

    **c.** second-hand smoke

    **d.** none of the above

6. The bicuspid valve controls blood flow between the _____.

    **a.** heart and lungs

    **b.** arteries and veins

    **c.** atrium and ventricle

    **d.** none of the above

7. A graft that uses skin from one's own body is a(n) _____.

    **a.** autograft

    **b.** allograft

    **c.** heterograft

    **d.** xenograft

8. The heart is located in the _____.

    **a.** abdominal cavity

    **b.** pelvic cavity

    **c.** thoracic cavity

    **d.** cranial cavity

9. Red blood cells are _____.

    **a.** neutrophils

    **b.** eosinophils

    **c.** basophils

    **d.** none of the above

10. A disease-causing agent is a(n) _____.

    **a.** pathogen

    **b.** macrophage

    **c.** antibody

    **d.** antitoxin

11. The system that secretes hormones is the _____.

    **a.** endocrine system

    **b.** cardiovascular system

    **c.** lymphatic system

    **d.** immune system

**12.** Nails are made of _____.

    **a.** lunula                            **c.** keratin

    **b.** cuticles                         **d.** adipose

**13.** The area of the spinal cord that affects the muscles of the legs is the _____.

    **a.** cervical                         **c.** brachial

    **b.** coccygeal                      **d.** sacral

**14.** An agent that induces sleep is a(n) _____.

    **a.** hypnotic                        **c.** anticonvulsant

    **b.** analgesic                       **d.** antibiotic

**15.** Urine travels from the ureters to the _____

    **a.** kidney                            **c.** meatus

    **b.** bladder                        **d.** glomerulus

**16.** A meningocele is associated with _____.

    **a.** Tay-Sachs                     **c.** hydrocephalus

    **b.** spina bifida                  **d.** concussion

**17.** An agent that causes the pupil to contract is a(n) _____.

    **a.** eye drop                       **c.** mydriatic

    **b.** miotic                           **d.** antiseptic

**18.** The oil-producing glands are the _____.

    **a.** sebaceous glands           **c.** sudoriferous glands

    **b.** sweat glands                **d.** apocrine glands

**19.** The epidermis includes the _____.

    **a.** stratified squamous epithelium     **c.** stratum germinativum

    **b.** stratum corneum             **d.** all of the above

**20.** Tendons are a type of _____.

    **a.** epithelial tissue         **c.** muscle tissue

    **b.** connective tissue       **d.** nervous tissue

**21.** HIV can be transmitted _____.

    **a.** during birth          **c.** in infected blood

    **b.** via sexual contact      **d.** all of the above

**22.** Metastasis means _____.

    **a.** a disease is localized     **c.** an anaphylactic reaction is taking place

    **b.** a disease has spread      **d.** none of the above

**23.** The alimentary canal includes the _____.

    **a.** appendix           **c.** liver

    **b.** esophagus         **d.** pancreas

**24.** An organ of the lymph system is the _____.

    **a.** lung            **c.** gallbladder

    **b.** spleen          **d.** pancreas

**25.** Chemotherapy is used to cause a _____.

    **a.** remission         **c.** recurrence

    **b.** relapse         **d.** none of the above

## Fill in the Blanks

Put the word that best completes the sentence in the space provided.

  **1.** Surgical removal of an embolus is a(n) _____.

  **2.** Agents that promote the removal of water are _____.

  **4.** A papule is a small, elevated _____.

  **5.** Blood vessel lesions that show through the skin are _____ lesions.

  **6.** A purified protein derivative of tuberculin is used in the _____ test.

  **7.** Any abnormal tissue growth is a(n) _____.

8. A hard, thickened area of skin is a(n) _____.

9. An inflammation of the pericardium is _____.

10. Ace inhibitors lower _____.

11. An antigen is injected between layers of skin in a(n) _____ test.

12. The excretion of sweat is called _____.

13. Rheumatologists treat disorders of the _____.

14. Joints are also called _____.

15. A skin graft from one's own body is a(n) _____.

16. Kaposi's sarcoma is often associated with _____.

17. A subcutaneous tissue infection is a(n) _____.

18. A frictional sound heard on auscultation is a(n) _____.

19. To prevent emboli, most surgical patients are given a(n) _____.

20. A sudden drop of blood supply to a vessel is a(n) _____.

21. Electrical impulses of the brain are recorded in an _____.

22. The creation of a surgical opening in the abdomen through which urine exits the body is a(n) _____.

23. A glomulerus is a group of _____.

24. Any disease of the blood with abnormal material present is a type of _____.

25. The hollow, muscular organ that stores urine is the _____.

26. Inhibin inhibits the production of _____.

27. The taste buds are contained in small raised areas of the tongue called _____.

28. The outer portion of each adrenal gland is the adrenal _____.

29. Lack of iodine in the diet can cause a(n) _____.

30. The prostate gland secretes _____.

31. The lingual tonsils are the two mounds of tissue at the back of the _____.

32. The cells in blood that destroy foreign substances are _____.

**33.** The most important male sex hormone is _____.

**34.** Plasma consists of 92 percent _____.

**35.** The area between the penis and anus is called the _____.

**36.** Inflammation of a ganglion is _____.

**37.** Damage to the cerebrum at or prior to birth causes _____.

**38.** Plaque in the wall of an artery is called a(n) _____.

**39.** All the sublayers of epidermis together are called stratifed squamous _____.

**40.** Carbon dioxide is a _____ product.

**41.** Bone-forming cells are _____.

**42.** Burning wounds to control bleeding is _____.

**43.** An agent that relieves pain is a(n) _____.

**44.** An open fracture is also called a _____ fracture.

**45.** Bone hardening depends on vitamin D, phosphorus, and _____.

**46.** An agent that adds oils to skin is a(n) _____.

**47.** The testes produce male hormones called _____.

**48.** Insulin is secreted by the islets of _____.

# CAM Review

**1.** In the space below, explain the difference between complementary and alternative medicine.

_____

_____

_____

_____

**2.** List the five classifications of CAM that the federal government currently recognizes.

   **a.** _____

   **b.** _____

c. _____

d. _____

**3.** Briefly describe the basis of naturopathy.

_____

_____

_____

_____

**4.** How does homeopathy differ from naturopathy?

_____

_____

_____

_____

**5.** Describe three manipulative and body-based methods.

a. _____

_____

b. _____

_____

c. _____

_____

# APPENDIX A

# Combining Forms, Prefixes, and Suffixes

Listed below are the combining forms, prefixes, and suffixes used in medical terminology. They are useful in building medical terms.

**a-, an-**  *prefix.* not, without, lacking.

**ab-**  *prefix.* from; away; off.

**abdomin-, abdomino-**  *combining form.* abdomen.

**acanth-**  *combining form.* thorny or having spines.

**acet-, aceto-**  *combining form.* two-carbon fragment of acetic acid.

**- acousis, -acusis -**  *suffix.* hearing.

**acro-**  *prefix.* **1.** end, tip, or peak. **2.** extremity.

**acromi-, acromio-**  *combining form.* the acromion.

**actin-, actino-**  *combining form.* ray, beam; having raylike structures.

**ad-**  *prefix.* to, toward, near the midline.

**-ad**  *suffix.* toward, in the direction of.

**aden-, adeno-**  *combining form.* gland or glandular.

**adipo-**  *combining form.* fat, fatty.

**adren-, adreno-, adrenal-, adrenalo-**  *combining form.* adrenal gland.

**aero-**  *combining form.* air.

**agglutin-, agglutino-**  *combining form.* adhere or combine.

**-al**  *suffix.* of or involving; process.

**algesio-**  *combining form.* pain.

**-algesia**  *suffix.* pain.

**-algia**  *suffix.* pain or a specific painful condition.

**algo-**  *combining form.* pain.

**allo-**  *prefix.* of the same species.

**alveol-, alveolo-**  *combining form.* alveolus.

**ambi-**  *combining form.* **1.** around, on all sides. **2.** both, double.

**amnio-**  *combining form.* amnion.

**an-¹**  *prefix.* not.

**an-², ana-**  *prefix.* up; upward: back; backward.

**andr-, andro-**  *combining form.* masculine.

**angi-, angio-**  *combining form.* blood or lymph vessel.

**aniso-**  *combining form.* not equal, disimilar.

**ankyl-, anklyo-**  *combining form.* fused; stiffened.

**ant-, anti-**  *prefix.* against, opposite.

**ante-**  *prefix.* **1.** before: *for example,* antepartum. **2.** in front of.

**antero-**  *prefix.* anterior.

**anthrac-, anthraco-**  *combining form.* coal; carbon; carbuncle.

**-apheresis**  *combining form.* removal, separation.

**apic-, apico-**  *combining form.* apex.

**apo-**  *prefix.* separated from; derived from.

**aponeur-, aponeuro-**  *combining form.* tendon-like.

**append-**  *combining form.* appendage, appendix.

**appendic-, appendico-**   *combining form.* appendix.
**arteri-, arterio-**   *combining form.* artery.
**arteriol-, arteriolo-**   *combining form.* arteriole.
**arthr-, arthro-**   *combining form.* joint.
**astro-**   *combining form.* star.
**-ate**   *suffix.* replaces "-ic" in acids after the acid has been neutralized, such as nitrate from nitric acid.
**ather-, athero-**   *combining form.* soft fatty deposit.
**atri-, atrio-**   *combining form.* atrium.
**audio-**   *combining form.* sound, hearing.
**aut-, auto-**   *combining form.* self, same.

**bacteri-, bacterio-**   *combining form.* bacteria.
**balan-, balano-**   *combining form.* glans penis.
**bar-, baro-**   *combining form.* weight, pressure.
**bas-, baso-**   *combining form.* base; foundation.
**bi-**   *prefix.* twice, double.
**bio-**   *combining form.* life, living.
**blast-, blasto-**   *combining form.* immature cell.
**-blast**   *suffix.* immature, forming.
**blephar-, blepharo-**   *combining form.* eyelid.
**brachi-, brachio-**   *combining form.* arm.
**brachy-**   *combining form.* short.
**brady-**   *combining form.* slow.
**bronch-, bronchi-, broncho-**   *combining form.* bronchus, bronchi.
**bronchiol-**   *combining form.* bronchiole.
**bucc-, bucco-**   *combining form.* cheek.
**burs-, burso-**   *combining form.* bursa, bursae.

**calcaneo-**   *combining form.* heel.
**calic-, calico-, calio-**   *combining form.* calyx.
**capno-**   *combining form.* carbon dioxide.
**carcin-, carcino-**   *combining form.* cancer.
**card-, cardi-, cardio-**   *combining form.* heart.
**-cardia**   *suffix.* the condition of having a specific kind of heart or heartbeat.
**carp-, carpo-**   *combining form.* wrist.
**cata-**   *prefix,* down.
**cec-, ceco-**   *combining form.* cecum.
**-cele**   *suffix.* **1.** tumor or swelling.. **2.** cavity.
**celio-**   *combining form.* abdomen.
**-centesis**   *suffix.* puncture.
**centi-**   *prefix.* one hundred.
**cephal-, cephalo-**   *combining form.* head.
**-cephaly**   *suffix.* head.
**cerebr-, cerebro-**   *combining form.* cerebrum.
**cervic-, cervico-**   *combining form.* neck.
**cheil-, cheilo-**   *combining form.* lips.
**chemo-**   *combining form.* chemical.
**chlor-, chloro-**   *combining form.* **1.** green. **2.** chlorine.
**chol-, chole-, cholo-**   *combining form.* bile.
**cholang-, cholangi-, cholangio-**   *combining form.* bile duct.
**cholecyst-, cholecysto-**   *combining form.* gallbladder.
**choledoch-, choledocho-**   *combining form.* the common bile duct.
**chondr-, chondro-**   *combining form.* cartilage.
**chorio-**   *combining form.* membrane, especially the chorion.
**chrom-, chromat-, chromo-**   *combining form.* color.
**chron-, chrono-**   *combining form.* time.

**chyl-, chylo-**  *combining form.* chyle.
**-cidal**  *suffix.* killing.
**-cide**  *suffix.* one that kills.
**cine-**  *combining form.* movement.
**circum-**  *prefix.* around.
**-clasis**  *suffix.* breaking.
**-clast**  *suffix.* breaking.
**cleido-**  *combining form.* clavicle.
**clino-**  *combining form.* sloping: curving.
**co-, com-, con-**  *prefix.* with, together.
**-coccus**  *suffix.* belonging to a group of bacteria having a spherical shape.
**cochle-, cochleo-**  *combining form.* of or relating to the inner ear.
**col-, colo-**  *combining form.* colon.
**colp-, colpo-**  *combining form.* vagina.
**com-**  *prefix.* with, together.
**con-**  *prefix.* with, together.
**condyl-**  *combining form.* rounded, knob-like, condyle.
**contra-**  *prefix.* opposed, against..
**cor-, core-, coreo-**  *combining form.* pupil.
**corne-, corneo-**  *combining form.* cornea.
**cortic-, cortico-**  *combining form.* cortex.
**cost-, costo-**  *combining form.* rib.
**counter-**  *prefix.* against.
**crani-, cranio-**  *combining form.* skull.
**-crine**  *suffix.* secreting.
**cryo-**  *combining form.* cold.
**crypt-, crypto-**  *combining form.* hidden or obscure.
**culdo-**  *combining form.* pouch.
**-cusis**  *suffix.* hearing.
**cyan-**  *combining form.* blue.
**cycl-, cyclo-**  *abbreviation.* circle; cycle; ciliary body.
**cyst-, cysto-**  *combining form.* **1.** the bladder. **2.** cyst.
**cyt-, cyto-**  *combining form.* a cell.
**-cyte**  *suffix.* a cell.

**dacryo-**  *combining form.* tear or tears; lacrymal sac or duct
**dacryocyst-, dacryocysto-**  *combining form.* of or involving the lacrimal sac.
**dactyl-, dactylo-**  *combining form.* fingers; toes.
**-dactyly**  *suffix.* the condition of have a specified kind or number of fingers or toes.
**de-**  *prefix.* away from.
**dent-, denti-**  *combining form.* teeth.
**derm-, derma-, dermo-**  *combining form.* skin.
**-derma**  *suffix.* skin.
**dermat-, dermato-**  *combining form.* skin.
**-desis**  *suffix.* binding.
**desm-, desmo-**  *combining form.* fibrous connection; ligament.
**dextr-, dextro-**  right.
**dextro-**  *combining form.* right; on the right side.
**di-**  *prefix.* two, twice.
**dia-**  *prefix.* through, throughout, completely.
**dipl-, diplo-**  *combining form.* double, two-fold.
**dips-, dipso-**  *combining form.* thirst.
**dis-**  *prefix.* in two, apart.
**dors-, dorsi-, dorso-**  *combining form.* back.
**dynamo-**  *combining form.* strength or force; energy.

**-dynia**   *suffix.* pain.
**dys-**   *prefix.* abnormal, difficult.

**echo-**   *combining form.* sound.
**-ectasia, -ectasis**   *suffix.* dilation, expansion.
**ecto-**   *combining form.* outer, on the outside.
**-ectomy**   *suffix.* excision, removal.
**ectro-**   *combining form.* missing (usually from birth).
**-edema**   *suffix.* swelling.
**electro-**   *combining form.* electrical.
**embryo-**   *combining form.* of or relating to an embryo.
**-emesis**   *suffix.* vomit.
**-emia**   *suffix.* blood.
**encephal-, encephalo-**   *combining form.* the brain.
**end-, endo-**   *combining form.* within, inner, absorbing, or containing.
**enter-, entero-**   *combining form.* intestines.
**epi-**   *prefix.* over.
**epididym-, epididymo-**   *combining form.* epididymis.
**episo-**   *combining form.* vulva.
**erythro-**   *combining form.* red, redness.
**esophag-, esophago-**   *combining form.* esophagus.
**-esthesia**   *suffix.* sensation, perception.
**eu-**   *prefix.* well, good, normal.
**exo-**   *prefix.* external, on the outside.
**extra-**   *prefix.* without, outside of.

**fasci-, fascio-**   *combining form.* a band of fibrous tissue.
**femor-, femoro-**   *combining form.* relating to the femur or thigh.
**-ferous**   *suffix.* carrying, yielding.
**fet-, feti-, feto-**   *combining form.* fetus
**fibr-, fibro-**   *combining form.* fiber.
**fibrin-, fibrino-**   *combining form.* fibrin.
**fluor-, fluoro-**   *combining form.* **1.** fluorine. **2.** fluorescence.
**-form**   *suffix.* having the form of.
**fung-, fungi-, fungo-**   *combining form.* fungus.

**galact-, galacto-**   *combining form.* milk.
**gameto-**   *combining form.* gamete.
**gangli-, ganglio-**   *combining form.* ganglion.
**gastr-, gastro-**   *combining form.* stomach.
**-gen**   *suffix.* precursor of.
**-genesis**   *suffix.* origin; production.
**-genic**   *suffix.* producing; generating.
**geno-**   *combining form.* gene, genetic.
**geronto-**   *combining form.* old age.
**gingiv-, gingivo-**   *combining form.* gum.
**gli-, glia-, glio-**   *combining form.* neuroglia.
**-globin**   *suffix.* protein.
**-globulin**   *suffix.* protein.
**gloss-, glosso-**   *combining form.* tongue.
**gluc-, gluco-**   *combining form.* glucose.
**glyc-, glyco-**   *combining form.* sugar, glycogen.
**gnatho-**   *combining form.* jaw.
**gonio-**   *combining form.* angle.
**-gram**   *suffix.* a written record.
**granul-, granulo-**   *combining form.* granule or granular.

**-graph**   *suffix.* instrument.
**gyne-, gynec-, gyneco-**   *combining form.* woman.

**hem-, hemo-**   *combining form.* blood.
**hemangi-, hemangio-**   *combining form.* blood vessel.
**hemat-, hemato-**   *combining form.* blood.
**hemi-**   *combining form.* half.
**hepat-, hepato-**   *combining form.* liver.
**hernio-**   *combining form.* hernia.
**hetero-**   *combining form.* other; different.
**hidr-, hidro-**   *combining for.* sweat; sweat glands.
**hist-, histo-**   *combining form.* body tissue.
**histi-, histio-**   *combining form.* body tissue, especially connective tissue.
**homeo-, homo-**   *combining form.* like; similar.
**hyal-**   *combining form.* glassy.
**hydr-, hydro-**   *combining form.* water, liquid.
**hymen-, hymeno-**   *combining form.* hymen.
**hyper-**   *prefix.* excessive or above normal.
**hypo-**   *prefix.* low, below normal.

**-ia**   *suffix.* condition; disease.
**-iasis**   *suffix.* pathological condition characterized or produced by.
**-ic**   *suffix.* of, pertaining to, relating to, or characterized by.
**ichthy-, ichthyo-**   *combining form.* fish or fishlike.
**-ics**   *suffix.* the science or study of.
**idio-**   *combining form.* unknown.
**ile-, ileo-**   *combining form.* ileum.
**immuno-**   *combining form.* immune; immunity.
**in-**   *prefix.* into or not.
**infra-**   *prefix.* inferior, below, or beneath.
**inter-**   *prefix.* between; within.
**intra-**   *prefix.* within.
**irid-, irido-**   *combining form.* iris of the eye.
**ischi-, ischio-**   *combining form.* ischium.
**-ism**   *suffix.* state or condition of.
**iso-**   *prefix.* equal; uniform.
**-itis**   *suffix.* inflammation or disease of.

**jejun-, jejuno-**   *combining form.* jejunum.

**karyo-**   *combining form.* nucleus.
**kerat-, kerato-**   *combining form.* **1.** the cornea. **2.** horny tissue or cells.
**ket-, keto-**   *combining form.* ketone or ketone group.
**-kinesia**   *suffix.* motion.
**-kinesis**   *suffix.* movement or activation.
**-kinetic**   *suffix.* of or relating to motion or movement.
**kyph-, kypho-**   *combining form.* abnormal curvature of the spine; hunchback.

**labi-, labio-**   *combining form.* lips.
**lact-, lacti-, lacto-**   *combining form.* milk.
**laparo-**   *combining form.* abdomen, abdominal wall.
**laryng-, laryngo-**   *combining form.* the larynx.
**later-, latero-**   *combining form.* side.
**leiomy-, leiomyo-**   *combining form.* smooth muscle.
**-lepsy**   *suffix.* seizure.
**lept-, lepto-**   *combining form.* thin, narrow, weak, delicate.

**-leptic**    *suffix.* a type of seizure.
**leuk-, leuko-**    *combining form.* white.
**levo-**    *combining form.* left.
**lip-, lipo-**    *combining form.* fat.
**lith-, litho-**    *combining form.* stone, calculus, calcification.
**-lith**    *suffix.* stone, calculus, calcification.
**-lithiasis**    *suffix.* stone formation or condition.
**lob-, lobo-**    *combining form.* lobe.
**-logy**    *suffix.* the science or study of.
**lumb-, lumbo-**    *combining form.* loins.
**lymph-, lympho-**    *combining form.* lymph.
**lymphaden-, lymphadeno-**    *combining form.* lymph node.
**-lytic**    *suffix.* involving or pertaining to lysis (of the matter or type specified).

**macro-**    *prefix.* large; long.
**mal-**    *prefix.* bad, ill; abnormal.
**-malacia**    *suffix.* softening.
**mamm-, mamma-, mammo-**    *combining form.* breast.
**-mania**    *suffix.* having an extreme compulsion for something.
**mast-, masto-**    *combining form.* breast.
**mastoid-, mastoido-**    *combining form.* breast.
**maxill-, maxillo-**    *combining form.* maxilla.
**meat-, meato-**    *combining form.* meatus.
**medi-, medio-**    *combining form.* middle; central.
**mediastin-, mediastino-**    *combining form.* mediastinum.
**megalo-**    *prefix.* **1.** very large; huge. **2.** abnormally large; enlarged.
**-megaly**    *suffix.* abnormal enlargement or growth.
**melan-, melano-**    *combining form.* melanin.
**-melia**    *suffix.* limb.
**mening-, meningi-, meningo-**    *combining form.* meninges; membrane,
**meno-**    *combining form.* menses; menstruation.
**mento-**    *combining form.* chin.
**mes-, meso-**    *combining form.* **1.** middle; central. **2.** intermediate; in between. **3.** mesentery.
**mesio-**    *combining form.* mesial.
**meta-**    *prefix.* after, behind, altered.
**-meter**    *suffix.* instrument for or method of measuring.
**metr-, metri-, metro-**    *prefix.* uterus.
**-metry**    *suffix.* process or method of measuring something.
**micro-**    *prefix.* meaning small.
**mid-**    *prefix.* middle.
**milli-**    *prefix.* one thousand, especially in the metric system.
**mon-, mono-**    *combining form.* involving one element or part; single; alone.
**-morph**    *suffix.* having a specified form or shape.
**morpho-**    *combining form.* form, shape, or structure.
**muc-, muci-, muco-**    *combining form.* mucus; mucous.
**multi-**    *prefix.* many.
**my-, myo-**    *prefix.* muscle.
**myc-, myco-**    *combining form.* fungus.
**myel-, myelo-**    *combining form.* **1.** bone marrow. **2.** the spinal cord and medulla oblongata. **3.** the myelin sheath enclosing nerve fibers.
**myo-**    *combining form.* muscle.
**myocardi, mycardio-**    *combining form.* myocardium.
**myx-, myxo-**    *combining form.* mucus.

**narc-, narco-**    *combining form.* numbness or drowsiness.
**nas-, naso-**    *combining form.* nose.

**necr-, necro-**   *combining form.* death or corpse.
**neo-**   *prefix.* new, recent.
**nephr-, nephro-**   *combining form.* kidney.
**neur-, neuri-, neuro-**   *combining form.* nerve, nervous system.
**noct-, nocti-, nocto-**   *combining form.* night.
**non-**   *prefix.* the reverse or opposite of something; not.
**norm-, normo-**   *combining form.* normal,
**nyct-, nycto-**   *combining form.* night.

**ocul-, oculo-**   *combining form.* eye.
**odont-, odonto-**   *combining form.* tooth, teeth.
**-odynia**   *suffix.* pain.
**-oid**   *suffix.* like, resembling.
**olig-, oligo-**   *combining form.* too few, too little; scanty.
**-oma** (*pl.* **-omas** or **-omata**)   *suffix.* tumor, neoplasm.
**oment-, omento-**   *combining form.* omentum.
**omphal-, omphalo-**   *combining form.* navel; umbilicus.
**onco-**   *combining form.* tumor, mass, swelling.
**onych-, onycho-**   *combinng form.* nail.
**oo-**   *combining form.* egg.
**oophor-, oophoro-**   *combining form.* ovary.
**ophthalm-, ophthalmo-**   *combining form.* eye.
**-opia**   *suffix.* vision.
**-opsia**   *suffix.* defect in vision or eyesight.
**-opsy**   *suffix.* examination; viewing; process of viewing.
**opt-, opto-**   *combining form.* vision.
**or-, oro-**   *combining form.* mouth.
**orch-, orchi-, orchid-, orchido-, orchio-**   *combining form.* testicle.
**organo-**   *combining form.* organ.
**orth-, ortho-**   *combining form.* straight, correct.
**-ose**   *suffix.* **1.** full of. **2.** carbohydrate.
**-osis**   *suffix.* condition; disorder.
**ost-, oste-, osteo-**   *combining form.* bone.
**ot-, oto-**   *combining form.* ear.
**-ous**   *suffix.* full of, possessing.
**ov-, ovi-, ovo-**   *combining form.* egg.
**ovari-, ovario-**   *combining form.* ovary.
**over-**   *prefix.* excessive; above normal.
**-oxia**   *suffix.* oxygen.
**oxy-**   *combining form.* 1. oxygen. 2. pointed.

**pachy-**   *combining form.* thick.
**palato-**   *combining form.* palate.
**pan-**   *prefix.* all; entire; the whole.
**pancreat-, pancreato-**   *combining form.* pancreas.
**par-, para-**   *prefix.* **1.** near; beside. **2.** beyond; outside. **3.** assistant; associate. **4.** abnormal.
**-para**   *suffix.* woman who has borne the indicated number of children.
**-parous**   *suffix.* giving birth to; bearing.
**-partum**   *suffix.* labor and childbirth.
**-pathic**   *suffix.* of or pertaining to disease.
**patho-**   *combining form.* disease.
**-pathy**   *suffix.* disease or diseased condition.
**ped-, pedi-, pedo-**   *combining form.* **1.** child. **2.** foot or feet.
**pelv-, pelvi-**   *combining form.* pelvis.
**-penia**   *suffix.* lack, deficiency.
**-pepsia**   *suffix.* digestion.

**per-**    *prefix.* **1.** through. **2.** intensely.

**peri-**    *prefix.* about, around, near.

**pericardi-, pericardio-**    *combining form.* near the heart; pericardium.

**perine-, perineo-**    *combining form.* perineum.

**peritone-, peritoneo-**    *combining form.* peritoneum.

**-pexy**    *suffix.* fixation; attachment.

**phac-, phaco-**    *combining form.* shaped like a lens; birthmark.

**-phag-, phago-**    *combining form.* consuming, eating.

**-phage, -phagia, -phagy**    *suffix.* consuming, eating.

**phalang-, phalango-**    *combining form.* finger, toe.

**pharmaco-**    *combining form.* drugs.

**-phasia**    *suffix.* speech disorder.

**-phil, -phile, -philic, -philia**    *suffix.* love; desire for.

**phleb-, phlebo-**    *combining form.* vein.

**-phobia**    *suffix.* fear.

**-phobic**    *suffix.* suffering from a phobia.

**phon-, phono-**    *combining form.* sound, voice.

**-phonia**    *suffix.* sound.

**-phoresis**    *suffix.* carrying, transmission.

**-phoria**    *suffix.* feeling.

**phot-, photo-**    *combining form.* light.

**phren-, phreno-**    *combining form.* diaphragm.

**-phrenia**    *suffix.* mental disorder.

**-phthisis**    *suffix.* wasting away, shriveling.

**-phylaxis**    *suffix.* protection.

**phyto-**    *combining form.* plant.

**-plakia**    *suffix.* plaque (small patch on skin).

**-plasia**    *suffix.* growth.

**-plasm**    *suffix.* tissue.

**-plastic**    *suffix.* forming.

**-plasty**    *suffix.* shaping, forming, repairing.

**-plegia**    *suffix.* paralysis.

**-plegic**    *suffix.* a person who is paralyzed.

**pleur-, pleuro-**    *combining form.* **1.** pleura. **2.** rib, side.

**-pnea**    *suffix.* breath.

**pneum-, pneuma-, pneumat-, pneumato-, pneumo-**    *combining form.* **1.** breath. **2.** air.

**pneumon-, pneumono-**    *combining form.* breath; lung.

**-poiesis**    *suffix.* formation, production.

**-poietic**    *suffix.* forming, producing.

**poikilo-**    *combining form.* varied, irregular.

**poly-**    *prefix.* many, much.

**-porosis**    *suffix.* lessening in density; thinning out.

**post-**    *prefix.* after, following.

**pre-**    *prefix.* before.

**pro-**    *prefix.* before, forward.

**proct-, procto-**    *combining form.* anus, rectum.

**prostate-, prostat-, prostato-**    *combining form,* prostate gland.

**pseud-, pseudo-**    *combining form.* false.

**psych-, psycho-**    *combining form.* mind.

**-ptosis**    *suffix.* falling down or sagging of an organ.

**pub-, pubo-**    *combining form.* pubic, pubis.

**pulmon-, pulmono-**    *combining form.* the lungs.

**pupill-, pupillo-**    *combining form.* pupil.

**py-, pyo-**    *combining form.* pus.

**pyel-, pyelo-**    *combining form.* pelvis.

**pylor-, pyloro-**    *combining form.* the pylorus (outlet of the stomach).

**quadri-**   *prefix.* four.

**rach-, rachi-, rachio-**   *combining form.* spine.
**radi-, radio-**   *combining form.* radiation.
**radicul-, radiculo-**   *combining form.* relating to the root, as of a nerve or tooth.
**re-**   *prefix.* **1.** again. **2.** backward.
**rect-, recto-**   *combining form.* rectum.
**ren-, reni-, reno-**   *combining form.* kidney.
**retic-, reticulo-**   *combining form.* network.
**retin-, retino-**   *combining form.* retina.
**retro-**   *prefix.* **1.** backward. **2.** located behind.
**rhabdomy-, rhabdomyo-**   *combining form.* striated muscle.
**rheumat-, rheumato-**   *combining form.* joint.
**rhin-, rhino-**   *combining form.* the nose, nasal.
**-rrhagia**   *suffix.* an excessive flow.
**-rrhaphy**   *suffix.* suture.
**-rrhea**   *suffix.* flow or discharge.
**-rrhexis**   *suffix.* rupture.

**sacr-, sacro-**   *combining form.* sacrum
**salping-, salpingi-, salpingo-**   *combining form.* salpinx.
**sarc-, sarco-**   *combining form.* flesh.
**-sarcoma**   *suffix.* a malignant tumor formed in connective tissues.
**-schisis**   *suffix.* splitting.
**schisto-**   *combining form.* split; cleft.
**schiz-, schizo-**   *combining form.* **1.** split; cleft: schizonychia. **2.** schizophrenia.
**scler-, sclero-**   *combining form.* **1.** hard. scleroderma. **2.** sclera.
**-sclerosis**   *suffix.* sclerosis.
**scoli-, scolio-**   *combining form.* twisted; curved.
**-scope**   *suffix.* an instrument used for viewing or examining.
**-scopy**   *suffix.* viewing; seeing; observing.
**scot-, scoto-**   *combining form.* darkness.
**semi-**   *prefix.* **1.** half; partial; similar to.
**-sepsis**   *suffix.* sepsis.
**septo-**   *combining form.* septum.
**sero-**   *combining form.* serum.
**sial-, sialo-**   *combining form.* saliva, salivary gland.
**sidero-**   *combining form.* iron.
**sigmoid-, sigmoido-**   *combining form.* sigmoid colon.
**sinsitr-, sinistro-**   *combining form.* left.
**sinus-, sinuso-**   *combining form.* sinus.
**socio-**   *combining form.* social.
**somat- somato-**   *combining form.* body.
**-some**   *suffix.* body.
**-somnia**   *suffix.* sleep
**sono-**   *combining form.* sound.
**-spasm**   *suffix.* spasm.
**sperm-, spermat-, spermato- spermo-**   *combining form.* sperm.
**sphen- spheno-**   *combining form.* wedge; wedge-shaped.
**spher-, sphero-**   *combining form.* sphere.
**sphygm-, sphygmo-**   *combining form.* pulse.
**spin-, spino-**   *combining form.* spine, spinous.
**spir-, spiro-**   *combining form.* respiration.
**splen- spleno-**   *combining form.* spleen.
**spondyl-, spondylo-**   *combining form.* vertebra, vertebrae.

**staphyl-, staphylo-**   *combining form.* **1.** relating to staphylococci. **2.** relating to the uvula (of the soft palate of the mouth).

**-stat**   *suffix.* implies something that prevents motion or change.

**steat-, steato-**   *combining form.* fat.

**-stenosis**   *suffix.* stenosis.

**stereo-**   *combining form.* solid; three-dimensional.

**stern-, sterno-**   *combining form.* sternum.

**stomat-, stomato-**   *combining form.* mouth; stoma.

**-stomy**   *suffix.* surgical opening in an organ or body part.

**strepto-**   *combining form.* streptococcus.

**styl-, stylo-**   *combining form.* styloid process.

**sub-**   *prefix.* **1.** below. **2.** secondary. **3.** subdivision. **4.** not completely, almost.

**super-**   *prefix.* **1.** above; upon. **2.** superior. **3.** exceeding. **4.** excessive. **5.** containing a large amount of a specific ingredient.

**supra-**   *prefix.* above; over: supracostal.

**syn-**   *prefix.* **1.** together; united. **2.** same; similar.

**synov-, synovo-**   *combining form.* synovial membrane.

**tachy-**   *prefix.* speedy; fast; rapid.

**tars-, tarso-**   *combining form.* tarsus.

**-taxy**   *suffix.* order; arrangement.

**tel-, tele-, telo-**   *combining form.* **1.** distant. **2.** end.

**ten-, teno-**   *combining form.* tendon.

**terat-, terato-**   *combining form.* grossly deformed fetus or part.

**tetr-, tetra-**   *combining form.* four.

**therm-, thermo-**   *combining form.* heat.

**thorac-, thoracico-, thoraco-**   *combining form.* chest or thorax.

**thromb-, thrombo-**   *combining form.* blood clot.

**thym-, thymo-**   *combining form.* thymus.

**thyr-, thyro-**   *combining form.* thyroid.

**thyroid-,**   *combining form.* the thyroid gland.

**tibi-, tibio-**   *combining form.* of or relating to the tibia.

**toco-**   *combining form.* childbirth or labor.

**-tome**   *suffix.* **1.** cutting instrument. **2.** part, segment.

**tomo-**   *combining form.* cutting.

**-tomy**   *suffix.* incision.

**-tonia**   *suffix.* pressure; tension.

**tono-**   *combining form.* tone; pressure; tension.

**tonsill-, tonsillo-**   *combining form.* tonsil.

**tox-, toxi-, toxic-, toxico-, toxo-**   *combining form.* poison.

**trache-, tracheo-**   *combining form.* trachea.

**trachel-, trachelo-**   *combining form.* neck, usually of the uterus; uterine cervix.

**trans-**   *prefix.* across; through.

**tri-**   *prefix.* three.

**trich-, tricho-**   *combining form.* hair; thread.

**-tripsy**   *suffix.* crushing; pulverizing.

**-trophic**   *suffix.* relating to nutrition.

**-trophy**   *suffix.* nutrition; growth.

**-tropia**   *suffix.* abnormal deviation of the eye from a normal line of vision.

**-tropic**   *suffix.* involuntary response of an organism to turn away from or toward a stimulus.

**-tropin**   *suffix.* hormone.

**tympan-, tympano-**   *combining form.* tympanum, eardrum.

**-ule**   *suffix.* little; small (form of the thing specified).

**ultra-**   *prefix.* **1.** beyond or outside the limits of (the thing indicated). **2.** to an excessive or extreme degree of (the thing indicated).

**un-**    *prefix.* not.
**uni-**    *prefix.* one; single.
**ur-, uro-**    *combining form.* **1.** urine; urinary tract; urination.
**-uresis**    *suffix.* **1.** urination. **2.** excretion in the urine (of the substance indicated).
**ureter-, uretero-**    *combining form.* ureter.
**urethr-, urethro-**    *combining form.* urethra.
**-uria**    *suffix.* urine.
**urin-, urino-**    *combining form.* urine.
**utero-**    *combining form.* uterus.
**uve-, uveo-**    *combining form.* uvea.
**uvul-, uvulo-**    *combining form.* uvula.

**vag-, vago-**    *combining form.* vagus nerve.
**vagin-, vagino-**    *combining form.* vagina.
**valvul-, valvulo-**    *combining form.* valve.
**varico-**    *combining form.* **1.** varix or varicosity. **2.** varicose.
**vas-, vaso-**    *combining form.* **1.** blood vessel. **2.** vessel. **3.** vas deferens.
**ven-, veni-, veno-**    *combining form.* vein.
**ventricul-, ventriculo-**    *combining form.* ventricle.
**-version**    *suffix.* turning (of the type specified).
**vertebr-, vertebro-**    *combining form.* vertebra or vertebrae.
**vesic-, vesico-**    *combining form.* **1.** bladder. **2.** blister.
**vir-, viro-**    *combining form.* virus.
**viscer-, viscero-**    *combining form.* viscera.
**vulv-, vulvo-**    *combining form.* vulva.

**xanth-, xantho-**    *combining form.* yellow.
**xeno-**    *combining form.* strange; foreign matter.
**xer-, xero-**    *combining form.* dryness.
**xiph-, xipho-**    *combining form.* sword-shaped.

**zoo-**    *combining form.* animal.
**zyg-, zygo-**    *combining form.* a union; a pair or yoke.
**-zygous**    *suffix.* of or relating to a zygote.
**zymo-**    *combining form.* fermentation; enzymes.

# Medical Errors and Abbreviations

Recently, medical abbreviations have been linked to some of the worst medical errors, particularly those involving wrong doses of medication. As a result, the Joint Commission on Accreditation of Hospital Organizations (JCAHO) has come up with a list of nine prohibited abbreviations plus several as recommended for elimination in medical communication. For the prohibited abbreviations, it is suggested that the full words be substituted. We use the symbol ▲ to indicate such abbreviations. Table A-1 shows the prohibited abbreviations, what they can be confused with, and what should be substituted. Table A-2 shows suggested replacements for abbreviations that have the potential to cause medical errors. JCAHO has also suggested that each healthcare organization come up with its own list of frequently used and potentially misunderstood abbreviations.

Table A-1. Prohibited Abbreviations

| Abbreviation | Potential Problem | Solution |
| --- | --- | --- |
| 1. U (for unit) | Mistaken as zero, four or cc. | Write or speak "unit" |
| 2. IU (for international unit) | Mistaken as IV (intravenous) or 10 (ten). | Write or speak "international unit" |
| 3. Q.D. (once daily) 4. Q.O.D. (every other day) | Mistaken for each other. The period after the Q can be mistaken for an "I" and the "O" can be mistaken for "I". | Write or speak "daily" and "every other day" |
| 5. Trailing zero (X.0 mg) [*Note: Prohibited only for medication-related notations*]; 6. Lack of leading zero (.X mg) | Decimal point is missed and dosage is either too large or too small. | Never write a zero by itself after a decimal point (X mg), and always use a zero before a decimal point (0.X mg) |
| 7. MS 8. $MSO_4$ 9. $MgSO_4$ | Can mean morphine sulfate or magnesium sulfate. Potentially confused for one another. | Write or speak "morphine sulfate" or "magnesium sulfate" |

Table A-2. Suggested Additional Abbreviations to Avoid.

| Abbreviation | Potential Problem | Solution |
|---|---|---|
| μg (for microgram) | Mistaken for mg (milligrams) resulting in one thousand-fold dosing overdose. | Write "mcg" or speak microgram |
| H.S. (for half-strength or Latin abbreviation for bedtime) | Mistaken for either half-strength or hour of sleep (at bedtime). q.H.S. mistaken for every hour. All can result in a dosing error. | Write out or speak "half-strength" or "at bedtime" |
| T.I.W. (for three times a week) | Mistaken for three times a day or twice weekly resulting in an overdose. | Write or speak "3 times weekly" or "three times weekly" |
| S.C. or S.Q. (for subcutaneous) | Mistaken as SL for sublingual, or "5 every." | Write or speak "Sub-Q," "subQ," or "subcutaneously" |
| D/C (for discharge) | Interpreted as discontinue whatever medications follow (typically discharge meds). | Write "discharge" |
| c.c. (for cubic centimeter) | Mistaken for U (units) when poorly written. | Write or speak "ml" for milliliters |
| A.S., A.D., A.U. (Latin abbreviation for left, right, or both ears) | Mistaken for OS, OD, and OU, etc.). | Write or speak "left ear," "right ear" or "both ears" |

Listed below are the medical abbreviations

**a**  1. ante. 2. area. 3. asymmetric. 4. artery.

**A**  1. adenine. 2. alanine. 3. as a subscript, used to refer to alveolar gas..

**AA, aa**  1. amino acid. 2. AA Alcoholics Anonymous (www.alcoholics-anonymous.org).

**AAA**  abdominal aortic aneurysm.

**AMA**  American Medical Association. (www.ama-assn.org).

**AAMA**  American Association of Medical Assistants (www.aama-ntl.org).

**AAMT**  American Association for Medical Transcription (www.aamt.org).

**A&P**  1. auscultation and percussion. 2. anterior and posterior.

**ABC**  airway, breathing, and circulation, used in cardiac life support.

**ABCD**  airway, breathing, circulation, and defibrillation, used in cardiac life support.

**ABCDE**  airway, breathing, circulation and cervical spine, disability, and exposure, used in advanced trauma life support.

**ABG**  arterial blood gas.

**ABR**  auditory brainstem response.

**ABR test**  auditory brainstem response test.

**a.c.**  Latin *ante cibum,* before meals.

**AC**  air conduction.

**ACE**  angiotensin-converting enzyme.

**ACE2**  angiotensin-converting enzyme 2.

**AcG, ac-g**  accelerator globulin.

**Ach**  acetylcholine.

**ACL**  anterior cruciate ligament.

**ACR**   American College of Radiology.

**ACTH**   adrenocorticotropic hormone.

**AD**   Alzheimer's disease.

**A.D.**   Latin *auris dextra*, right ear.

**ADA**   **1.** American Dental Association (www.ada.org). **2.** Americans With Disabilities Act.

**ADAA**   American Dental Assistants Association (www.dentalassistants.org).

**ADD**   attention deficit disorder.

**ADH**   antidiuretic hormone.

**ADHD**   attention deficit hyperactivity disorder.

**ADLs**   activities of daily living.

**ad lib.**   Latin *ad libitum*, freely.

**Adm**   admission.

**ADR**   adverse drug reaction.

**AF**   atrial fibrillation

**AFB**   acid-fast bacillus.

**AFO**   ankle-foot orthotic.

**Ag**   Silver.

**A/G**   albumin:globulin ratio.

**AGN**   **1.** acute glomerulonephritis. **2.** acute necrotizing gingivitis.

**AHD**   atherosclerotic heart disease.

**AHIMA**   American Health Information Management Association (www.ahima.org).

**AI**   aortic insufficiency.

**AID**   artificial insemination by donor.

**AIDS** /ādz/   acquired immunodeficiency syndrome or acquired immunodeficiency disease.

**AIH**   artificial insemination, homologous (using the husband's semen).

**AK**   actinic keratosis.

**A-K**   above-the-knee.

**AKA**   above-the-knee amputation.

**ALL**   acute lymphoblastic leukemia; acute lymphocytic leukemia.

**ALS**   amyotrophic lateral sclerosis.

**ALT**   alanine aminotransferase.

**a.m., AM**   Latin *ante meridiem*, before noon.

**AMA**   American Medical Association (www.ama-assn.org).

**AMC**   arthrogryposis multiplex congenita.

**AML**   acute myelogenous lymphocytic leukemia; acute myeloblastic leukemia; acute myelocytic leukemia; acute myeloid leukemia.

**ANA**   antinuclear antibody titer, elevated in connective tissue disease.

**ANUG**   acute necrotizing ulcerative gingivitis.

**AP**   **1.** angina pectoris. **2.** arterial pressure. **3.** anterior pituitary. **4.** anteroposterior.

**AP & LAT**   anteposterior and lateral.

**APC**   **1.** acetylsalicylic acid, phenacetin, and caffeine, combined to make an analgesic. **2.** antigen-presenting cells.

**APTT**   activated partial thromboplastin time.

**AP view**   anteroposterior view.

**aq.**   water.

**ARB**   angiotensin II receptor blocker.

**ARC**   AIDS-related complex.

**ARDS**   adult respiratory distress syndrome or acute respiratory distress syndrome.

**ARF**   **1.** acute renal failure. **2.** acute respiratory failure.

**Arg**   arginine.

**AROM**   active range of motion.

**ART**   **1.** antiretroviral therapy. **2.** assisted reproductive technology.

**A.S.**   Latin *auris sinister*, left ear.

**ASA**   (drug caution code) abbreviation of acetylsalycylic acid (aspirin), placed on the label of a medication as a warning that it contains acytylsalysylic acid, which can cause complications for someone with specific medical conditions.

**ASD**   atrial septal defect.

**ASL**   American Sign Language.

**ASP**   aspartic acid.

AST   aspartate aminotransferase.

ATL   adult T-cell leukemia, adult T-cell leukemia/lymphoma, or adult T-cell lymphoma.

ATP   adenosine triphosphatase.

⚠ A.U.   Latin *auris unitas,* both ears.

AUL   acute undifferentiated leukemia.

AV   atrioventricular.

AVM   arteriovenous malformation.

AZT   azidothymadine, also known as zidovudine, a drug used in the treatment of HIV.


Ba   Barium.

BaE, Ba enema, BE   barium enema.

BAEP   brainstem auditory evoked potentials.

BAER   brainstem auditory evoked response.

BBB   blood-brain barrier.

BC   bone conduction.

BCG   bacillus of Calmette and Guerin (vaccination for tuberculosis).

BIA   biological impedance analysis.

b.i.d., bid, BID   Latin *bis in die,* two times a day (on prescriptions).

B-K   below the knee.

BKA   below-knee amputation.

BM   bowel movement.

BMD   bone mass density or bone mineral density.

BMI   body mass index.

BMR   basal metabolic rate.

BP, bp   blood pressure.

BPH   benign prostatic hyperplasia or benign prostatic hypertrophy.

BSA   body surface area.

BSE   bovine spongiform encephalopathy.

BUN   blood urea nitrogen.

bx, BX, Bx, Bx.   biopsy.

BZD   benzodiazepine.


C   **1.** calorie (kilocalorie). **2.** carbon. **3.** Celsius/centigrade. **4.** cervical vertebra/vertebrae. **5.** cytosine.

c   **1.** small calorie (gram calorie). **2.** centi-. **3.** curie.

Ca   calcium.

CA   **1.** (also **ca**) cancer/carcinoma. **2.** chronological age. **3.** coronary artery.

CA-125   cancer antigen 125.

CABG   coronary artery bypass graft.

CAD   coronary artery disease.

CAM   complementary and alternative medicine.

cap   capsule.

CAPD   continuous ambulatory peritoneal dialysis.

CAT   computerized axial tomography.

Cath, cath   catheter.

CBC   complete blood count.

CBT   cognitive behavioral therapy.

⚠ cc   cubic centimeter.

CCS   certified coding specialist (hospital).

CCS-P   certified coding specialist—physician.

CCU   coronary care unit.

CDA   certified dental assistant.

CDC   Centers for Disease Control and Prevention.

CEA   carcinoembryonic antigen.

CHF   congestive heart failure.

CIC   completely in the canal (said of hearing aids).

CIS   carcinoma in situ.

CJD   Creutzfeldt-Jakob's disease

**CK**   creatinine kinase.
**Cl**   chlorine.
**CLL**   chronic lymphocytic leukemia.
**Cm**   centimeter.
**CMA**   certified medical assistant.
**CMI**   cell-mediated immunity.
**CML**   chronic myelogenous leukemia.
**CMS**   Centers for Medicare and Medicaid Services (www.cms.gov).
**CMT**   certified medical transcriptionist.
**CMV**   cytomegalovirus.
**CNS**   central nervous system
**CO**   carbon monoxide.
**CO₂**   carbon dioxide.
**CoA**   coactation of the aorta.
**COBRA** /kō′brə/   U.S. federal Consolidated Omnibus Budget Reconciliation Act.
**COLD**   chronic obstructive lung disease.
**COPD**   chronic obstructive pulmonary disease.
**CP**   cerebral palsy.
**CPAP**   continuous positive airway pressure.
**CPC**   certified professional coder.
**CPC-H**   certified profession coder hospital.
**CPD**   cephalopelvic disproportion.
**CPK**   creatine phosphokinase.
**CPR**   cardiopulmonary resuscitation.
**CPT**   Current Procedural Terminology.
**CRF**   corticotropin-releasing factor.
**CRH**   corticotropin-releasing horomone.
**CRNA**   Certified Registered Nurse Anesthetist.
**CRP**   cAMP receptor protein; C-reactive protein.
**CSF**   cerebrospinal fluid.
**CSF**   colony-stimulating factor.
**CT**   computed tomography.
**CTS**   carpal tunnel syndrome.
**CVA**   cerebrovascular attack; cerebrovascular accident.
**CVC**   central venous catheter.
**CVD**   cardiovascular disease.
**CVP**   central venous pressure.
**CXR**   chest x-ray.

**D**   (drug caution code) found on the label of some medication, indicating that it may cause drowsiness.
**D & C, D and C**   dilation and curettage.
**D & E**   dilation and evacuation.
**dB**   decibel.
**DC**   1. (also **d.c.**) direct current. 2. Doctor of Chiropractic.
**DDS**   1. Doctor of Dental Surgery. 2. Denver Developmental Screening Test.
**def, DEF**   decayed, extracted, and filled, said of teeth.
**DES**   diethylstilbestrol.
**DEXA** scan /dĕk′sə/   the image or data produced by a special x-ray machine, used to measure bone density.
   [*d*ual-*e*nergy *x*-ray *a*bsorptiometry].
**DHEA**   dehydroepiandrosterone.
**DHF**   dengue hemorrhagic fever.
**DI**   diabetes insipidus.
**diff**   differential
**diff dx**   differential diagnosis.
**DLE**   discoid lupus erythematosus.
**DNA**   deoxyribonucleic acid.
**DNR**   do not resuscitate.

**D.O.**   Doctor of Osteopathy.

**DOA**   dead on arrival.

**Dr, Dr.**   doctor.

**DRE**   digital rectal exam.

**DRG**   diagnosis-related group, payment categories used by hospitals to charge fees to insurers.

**DRI**   dietary reference intake.

**DSA**   digital subtraction angiography.

**DSM**   *Diagnostic and Statistical Manual.*

**DT**   **1.** duration tetany, the spasm of degenerated muscle upon application of electrical current. **2.** diphtheria tetanus, a vaccine used for immunization of diphtheria and tetanus.

**DTs**   delirium tremens.

**DV**   daily value, as the recommended intake of a nutrient.

**DVT**   deep vein thrombosis.

**dx, DX**   diagnosis.

**DXA**   dual x-ray absorptiometry.

**EBCT**   electron beam computerized tomography.

**EBV**   Epstein-Barr virus.

**ECG, EKG**   electrocardiogram.

**ECHO** /ĕk′ō/   echocardiogram.

**ECMO** /ĕk′mō/   extracorporeal-membrane oxygenation, a complex therapeutic tool used in extreme ICU conditions where lung function has failed but is expected to recover within a few days.

**ECT**   electroconvulsive therapy; electroshock therapy.

**ED**   **1.** effective dose. **2.** emergency department. **3.** erectile dysfunction.

**EDC**   estimated date of confinement.

**EEE**   eastern equine encephalitis.

**EEG**   electroencephalogram.

**EENT**   eye, ear, nose, and throat. *See also* ENT.

**EF**   ejection fraction.

**EGD**   esophagogastroduodenoscopy.

**EIA**   enzyme immunoassay.

**EKG, ECG**   electrocardiogram.

**ELISA** /ĭ lī′zə, ĭ lĭs′ə/   enzyme-linked immunosorbent assay.

**elix.**   elixir.

**EMG**   electromyogram.

**EMR**   electronic medical record.

**EMT**   emergency medical technician.

**ENT**   ear, nose, throat. *See also* EENT.

**EPO**   erythropoietin.

**ER**   **1.** emergency room. **2.** estrogen receptor.

**ERCP**   endoscopic retrograde cholangiopancreatography.

**ERT**   estrogen replacement therapy.

**ESP**   extrasensory perception

**ESR**   erythrocyte sedimentation rate.

**ESRD**   end-stage renal disease.

**ESWL**   extracorporeal shock wave lithotripsy.

**F**   Fahrenheit.

**FAE**   fetal alcohol effects.

**FAP**   **1.** familial adenomatous polyposis. **2.** functional ambulation profile (analysis of a patient's ability to walk).

**FAS**   fetal alcohol syndrome.

**FBS**   fasting blood sugar.

**FBG**   fasting blood glucose.

**FDA**   Food and Drug Administration (www.fda.gov).

**FEF**   forced expiratory flow

**FET**   forced expiratory time.

**FEV₁**   forced expiratory volume measured during first second of expiration, useful in quantifying pulmonary disability.

**FHR**   fetal heart rate.

**FHT**   fetal heart tone.

**fMRI**   functional magnetic resonance imaging, a type of magnetic resonance imaging that demonstrates the correlation between physical changes and mental functioning.

**FNA**   fine needle aspiration biopsy.

**FP**   **1.** freezing point. **2.** family physician. **3.** family practice.

**ft.**   foot; feet.

**FTT**   failure to thrive.

**FUO**   fever of unknown origin.

**FVC**   forced vital capacity.

**G**   **1.** (drug caution code) abbreviation of glaucoma, placed on the label of a medication as a warning that it can cause complications for s omeone with the disease. **2.** gravida.

**g**   gram; grams.

**GB**   gallbladder

**GC**   gas chromatography.

**g-cal**   gram calorie.

**G-CSF**   granulocyte colony-stimulating factor.

**GDM**   gestational diabetes mellitus

**GERD** /gûrd/   gastroesophageal reflux disease.

**GH**   growth hormone.

**GHB**   gamma hydroxybutyrate

**GHz**   gigahertz gigahertzes.

**GI**   gastrointestinal.

**GI series**   gastrointestinal series.

**GI tract**   gastrointestinal tract.

**GIFT** /gĭft/   *abbreviation.* gamete intrafallopian transfer.

**GLC**   gas-liquid chromatography

**gm.**   gram; grams.

**GM-CSF**   granulocyte-macrophage colony-stimulating factor.

**GOT**   glutamic-oxaloacetic transaminase.

**gtt**   Latin *guttae*, drops.

**GSR**   galvanic skin response.

**GTT**   glucose tolerance test.

**GU**   genitourinary.

**Gy**   gray.

**GYN**   gynecology; gynecologist.

**H**   **1.** hyperopia; hyperopic. **2.** hydrogen. **3.** (drug caution code) found on the label of medication indicating that it can be habit forming.

**h**   **1.** height. **2.** hour.

**H&P**   history and physical.

**HAV**   hepatitis A virus, the RNA virus that causes hepatitis A.

**HB**   hepatitis B vaccine.

**Hb**   hemoglobin.

**HBIG**   hepatitis B immune globulin.

**HBV**   hepatitis B virus, the DNA virus that causes hepatitis B.

**HCFA**   Health Care Finance Administration, now the Centers for Medicare and Medicaid Services.

**HCG, HCG**   human chorionic gonadotropin.

**hct, HCT**   hematocrit.

**HCV**   hepatitis C virus, the RNA virus that causes hepatitus C.

**HD**   Hodgkin's disease.

**HDL**   high-density lipoprotein.

**HDN**   hemolytic disease of the newborn.

**HDV**   hepatitis D virus, the RNA virus that causes hepatitis D.

**HEV**   hepatitis E virus, the RNA virus that causes hepatitis E.

**Hg**   mercury.

**HGB, Hgb, HB**   hemoglobin.
**HGH**   human growth hormone
**HHS**   U.S. Department of Health and Human Services (www.hhs.gov).
**HIPAA**   Health Insurance Portability and Accountability Act.
**His**   histidine.
**HIV**   human immunodeficiency virus.
**HMD**   hyaline membrane disease.
**HMO**   health maintenance organization.
**H&P**   history and physical.
**HPV**   human papillomavirus.
**HRR**   high-risk register
**HRT**   hormone replacement therapy.
**HSG**   hysterosalpingography.
**HSV**   herpes simplex virus.
**HTLV**   human T-cell leukemia virus.
**HTN**   hypertension.
**Hz**   hertz.

**I**   (drug caution code) a symbol placed on the label of a medication, indicating possible adverse interaction if taken with other drugs.
**IBD**   inflammatory bowel disease.
**IBS**   irritable bowel syndrome.
**ICD-9-CM**   title of *International Classification of Diseases, 9th Revision, Clinical Modification*; system for diagnosis classification now in use for medical coding. ICD-10 is under review and expected to be adopted by 2010.
**ICF**   **1.** intermediate care facility. **2.** intracellular acid
**ICP**   intracranial pressure.
**ICU**   intensive care unit.
**IDDM**   insulin-dependant diabetes mellitus.
**Ig**   immunoglobulin.
**IgA**   immunoglobulin A.
**IgD**   immunoglobulin D.
**IgE**   immunoglobulin E.
**IGF**   insulin-like growth factor(s).
**IgG**   immunoglobulin G.
**IgM**   immunoglobulin M.
**IL**   interleukin
**IM**   intramuscular.
**IOL**   intraocular lens.
**IOP**   intraocular pressure.
**IPPB**   intermittent positive pressure breathing
**IPPV**   intermittent positive pressure ventilation
**IPV**   inactivated polio vaccine.
**IQ**   intelligence quotient.
**IU**   international unit
**IUD**   intrauterine contraceptive device.
**IUI**   intrauterine insemination.
**IV**   *adj.* **1.** intravenous. *n.* **2.** intravenous injection. **3.** intravenous drip.
**IVF**   in vitro fertilization.
**IVP**   intravenous pyelogram.

**JCAHO**   Joint Commission on Accreditation of Healthcare Organizations, an organization that inspects hospitals and reviews and gives accreditation to healthcare organizations (www.jcaho.org).

**K**   potassium.
**kg**   kilogram; kilograms.
**KUB**   kidneys, ureter, and bladder.

**l, L**   **1.** liter; liters. **2.** left.

**LASIK** /lā′sĭk/   laser-assisted in situ keratomileusis.

**lb.**   pound; pounds.

**LD**   lethal dose, often LD50 or LD95 to describe the dose at which 50% or 95% of the subjects (usually lab animals) die.

**LDH**   lactate dehydrogenase.

**LDL**   low-density lipoprotein.

**LE**   **1.** left eye (usually abreviated OS or o.s.). **2.** lupus erythematosus (usually abbreviated SLE)

**LEEP** /lēp/   loop electrosurgical excision procedure.

**LES**   lower esophageal sphincter.

**LFT**   liver function test.

**LI**   large intestine.

**LLQ**   left lower quadrant

**LP**   **1.** latency period. **2.** lipoprotein/low protein. **3.** lumbar puncture.

**LPN**   licensed practical nurse.

**LR**   **1.** labor room. **2.** lactated Ringer's (injection or solution). **3.** lateral rectus. **4.** light reaction or light reflex.

**LRM**   left radical mastectomy.

**LRT**   lower respiratory tract.

**LS**   **1.** left side. **2.** liver and spleen. **3.** lumbosacral. **4.** lymphosarcoma.

**LSH**   lutein-stimulating hormone.

**LTC**   long-term care.

**LUL**   **1.** left upper limb. **2.** left upper lobe (of lung).

**LUQ**   left upper quadrant.

**LV**   **1.** left ventricle. **2.** leukemia virus. **3.** live virus.

**LVAD**   left ventricular assist device

**LVN**   licensed vocational/visiting nurse.

**LVRS**   lung volume reduction surgery.

**Lys**   lysine.


**Mb**   myoglobin.

**MBC**   maximum breathing capacity.

**mcg**   microgram; micrograms.

**MCH**   **1.** mean corpuscular hemoglobin. **2.** maternal and child health (services).

**MCHC**   mean corpuscular hemoglobin concentration.

**MCP**   Metacarpophalangeal

**MCS**   multiple chemical sensitivity.

**MCV**   mean corpuscular volume.

**MD**   **1.** (*also* M.D.) Doctor of Medicine. **2.** muscular dystrophy.

**MDI**   metered-dose inhaler.

**ME**   medical examiner.

**MEP**   maximum expiratory pressure.

**MET**   **1.** metabolic equivalent. **2.** muscle energy technique.

**mets**   metastasis.

**mg**   milligram.

**MG**   myasthenia gravis.

**Mg**   magnesium

**mGy**   milligray.

**mh**   megahertz.

**MHz**   megahertz.

**MI**   **1.** myocardial infarction. **2.** mitral incompetence or inadequacy.

**MIS**   medical information system.

**ml, mL**   milliliter; milliliters.

**mm**   millimeter; millimeters.

**MMPI**   Minnesota Multiphasic Personality Inventory.

**Mn**   Manganese

**MP**   mentoposterior position.

**MPD**   **1.** multiple personality disorder. **2.** medical program director.

**MR**  mitral regurgitation.
**MRA**  magnetic resonance angiography.
**MRI**  magnetic resonance imaging.
**MS**  **1.** multiple sclerosis. **2.** mitral stenosis.
**MUGA** /mōō′gə/  multiple-gated acquisition scan.
**MVP**  mitral valve prolapse.

**N**  nitrogen.
**Na**  sodium.
**NARP**  neuropathy, ataxia, and retinitis pigmentosa, a genetic disease inherited from the mother, featuring weakness of the muscles near the trunk, ataxia (wobbliness), seizure, disease of the retina, and sometimes retardation or developmental delay.
**ND**  Doctor of Naturopathic Medicine.
**NEC**  not elsewhere classified (used in medical coding).
**neg, neg.**  negative.
**NG**  nasogastric.
**NHL**  non-Hodgkin lymphoma.
**NICU**  neonatal intensive care unit.
**NIDDM**  non-insulin-dependant diabetes mellitus.
**NK cell**  natural killer cell.
**NMR**  nuclear magnetic resonance.
**noc.**  Latin *nocte,* at night.
**noc, n.o.c.**  not otherwise classified.
**NOS**  not otherwise specified (used in medical coding).
**NPC**  Niemann-Pick's disease
**NPO, n.p.o.**  Latin *nil per os,* nothing by mouth.
**NREM sleep** /ĕn′rĕm′/ or **nonREM sleep** /nŏn′rĕm′/  non-rapid eye movement sleep.
**NSAID**  nonsteroidal anti-inflammatory drug.
**NTD**  neural tube defect.

**O$_2$**  oxygen.
**OB**  obstetrics; obstetrician.
**OB/GYN**  obstetrics and gynecology.
**OBS**  organic brain syndrome.
**OCD**  obsessive-compulsive disorder.
**OD**  **1.** *n.* an overdose. **2.** *v.* to overdose.
**o.d.**  Latin *oculus dexter,* the right eye (in optometry).
**oint, oint.**  ointment.
**OR**  operating room.
**orth**  orthopedic surgeon.
**OS, o.s.**  Latin *oculus sinister,* the left eye (in optometry).
**OSA**  obstructive sleep apnea.
**OSHA**  Occupation Safety and Health Administration (www.osha.gov).
**OT**  occupational therapy; occupational therapist.
**OTC**  over-the-counter (for sale without a prescription).
**OU, o.u.**  Latin *oculus uterque,* each eye (in prescriptions)
**oz, oz.**  ounce; ounces.

**PA**  **1.** physician assistant. **2.** posteroanterior (as in a typical chest x-ray). **3.** pulmonary artery.
**PAC**  premature atrial contraction.
**PACU** /păk′yōō′/  post-anesthesia care unit.
**Pap** /păp/  **1.** Papanicolaou('s). **2.** (*also* **pap**) Pap test. **3.** (*also* **pap**) Pap smear.
**PAP**  **1.** positive airway pressure. **2.** pulmonary artery pressure.
**Pb**  lead.
**p.c.**  Latin *post cibum,* after meals.
**PCA**  **1.** patient-controlled analgesia. **2.** posterior cerebral artery.
**PCL**  posterior cruciate ligament.

**PCP**   1. *Pneumocystis carinii* pneumonia. 2. primary care physician; primary care provider.
**PCR**   polymerase chain reaction, commonly used in medical testing to amplify particular sequences of DNA.
**PCT**   patient care technician.
**PCV**   packed cell volume.
**PD**   peritoneal dialysis.
**PDR**   1. *Physicians' Desk Reference.* 2. primary drug resistance.
**PDT**   photodynamic therapy.
**PE**   1. physical examination. 2. pleural effusion. 3. pulmonary edema. 4. pulmonary embolism.
**PED**   pediatric emergency department.
**peds**   pediatrics.
**PEEP**   positive end-expiratory pressure.
**PEFR**   peak expiratory flow rate.
**PEG**   percutaneous endoscopic gastrostomy.
**PERRL** or **PERRLA**   pupils equally round and reactive to light or pupils equally round and reactive to light and accommodation.
**PET** /pĕt/   positron emission tomography.
**PFT**   pulmonary function test.
**PICU**   pediatric intensive care unit.
**PID**   pelvic inflammatory disease.
**PIP**   proximal interphalangeal joints.
**PKD**   polycystic kidney disease.
**PKU**   phenylketonuria.
**PLT**   platelet count.
**PM, p.m.**   Latin *post meridian,* at night.
**PMS**   premenstrual syndrome.
**PN**   parenteral nutrition.
**PNS**   peripheral nervous system.
**p.o., PO**   Latin *per os,* by mouth.
**polio** /pō′lē ō′/   poliomyelitis.
**POS**   point of service.
**PPD**   1. postpartum depression. 2. purified protein derivative, used in a skin test for tuberculosis.
**PPMA**   postpolio muscular atrophy.
**PPO**   preferred provider organization.
**PPS**   postpolio syndrome.
**PR**   per rectum.
**PRBC**   packed red blood cells.
**preop** /prē′ŏp′/   preoperative.
**primip** /prī′mĭp, prī mĭp′/   primipara.
**PRK**   photorefractive keratectomy.
**PRN, p.r.n.**   Latin *pro re nata,* as needed (in prescriptions).
**PROM**   passive range of motion
**PSA**   prostate-specific antigen, a protein produced by the prostate gland that is used in the diagnosis of prostate cancer.
**PSG**   polysonmography
**pt**   patient.
**PT**   1. physical therapy. 2. physical therapist. 3. prothrombin time.
**Pl**   platinum.
**PTA**   percutaneous transluminal angioplasty.
**PTCA**   percutaneous transluminal coronary angioplasty.
**PTSD**   posttraumatic stress disorder.
**PTT**   partial thromboplastin time.
**PUBS**   percutaneous umbilical blood sampling, a technique used for diagnosing and treating a fetus in which a blood sample is taken from the umbilical vein by inserting a needle through the mother's abdominal and uterine walls.
**PUD**   peptic ulcer disease.
**pulv.**   powder (used in prescriptions).
**PUVA**   psoralen and UVA, a treatment for psoriasis that combines the medication psoralen with carefully timed UVA (ultraviolet light of A wavelength) exposure.

**PV**  **1.** polycythemia vera. **2.** peripheral vascular.
**PVC**  premature ventricular contraction.
**PVD**  peripheral vascular disease.
**PVS**  persistent vegetative state.

**q, q.**  every.
**qam, q.a.m.**  every morning.
**q.d., qd**  Latin *quaque die,* every day.
**q.h., qh**  Latin *quaque hora,* every hour.
**q.2h.**  every 2 hours.
**q.3h.**  every 3 hours.
**q.i.d., qid**  Latin *quatuor in die,* four times a day.
**q.n.s., QNS**  quantity not sufficient; used by a laboratory when an insufficient amount of specimen is received to perform a requested test.
**qod, q.o.d.**  every other day.
**qoh, q.o.h.**  every other hour.
**qpm, q.p.m.**  every evening.
**q.s., QS**  quantity sufficient; quantity required.
**qt**  **1.** (*also* **qt.**) quart; quarts. **2.** interval in QRS complex.

**R, r**  roentgen.
**Ra**  radium
**RA**  rheumatoid arthritis.
**rad** /răd/  radiation absorbed dose.
**RAST** /răst/  radioallergosorbent test.
**RBC**  **1.** red blood cells. **2.** red blood count.
**RD**  registered dietitian.
**RDA**  Recommended Daily Allowance; Recommended Dietary Allowance.
**RDS**  respiratory distress syndrome.
**rehab** /rē'hăb/  rehabilitation.
**REM** /rĕm/  rapid eye movements.
**RF**  rheumatoid factor.
**RIA**  radioimmunoassay.
**RLL**  right lower lobe.
**RLQ**  right lower quadrant.
**RMSF**  Rocky Mountain spotted fever.
**Rn**  radon.
**RN**  registered nurse.
**RNA**  ribonucleic acid.
**RP**  retinitis pigmentosa.
**RT, rt**  **1.** radiologic technologist. **2.** reaction time. **3.** recreational therapy. **4.** respiratory therapist.
**RUQ**  right upper quadrant.
**RV**  **1.** residual volume. **2.** right ventricle
**Rx, RX**  medical prescription.

**S**  sulfur.
**SA**  sinoatrial.
**SAD**  seasonal affective disorder.
**SA node**  sinoatrial node, the natural pacemaker of the heart.
**SARS** /särz/  severe acute respiratory syndrome.
**SBC**  systolic blood pressure.
**SBS**  shaken baby syndrome.
**sc, SC**  subcutaneous.
**Sc**  scandium.
**Se**  selenium.
**SERM**  selective estrogen receptor modulator.
**SGOT**  serum glutamic oxaloacetic transaminase.

**SGPT**   serum glutamic pyruvic transaminase.

**SIADH**   syndrome of inappropriate ADH (antidiuretic hormone).

**SIDS** /sĭdz/   sudden infant death syndrome.

**SL**   sublingual.

**SLE**   systemic lupus erythematosus.

**SLS**   Sjogren-Larsson's syndrome.

**SNOMED** /snō′mĕd′/   abbreviation. Systematized Nomenclature of Medical Terms, an international standardized system of medical terminology gradually being instituted worldwide.

**SOB**   shortness of breath.

**sol, sol.**   solution.

**SPECT**   single photon emission computed tomography.

**SPF**   sun protection factor.

▲ **sq**   subcutaneous.

**Sr**   strontium.

**SR**   **1.** sedimentation rate. **2.** sinus rhythm.

**SSPE**   subacute sclerosing panencephalitis.

**SSRI**   selective serotonin reuptake inhibitor.

**STD**   sexually transmitted disease.

**STH**   somatrophic hormone

**STI**   sexually transmitted infection.

**STM**   short-term memory.

**strep** /strĕp/   streptococcus.

**supp.**   supplement.

**susp.**   suspension.

**syr.**   syrup.

**sz**   seizure.


**T**   **1.** thymine. **2.** temperature. **3.** time. **4.** tablespoon; tablespoons.

**t.**   teaspoon; teaspoons.

**T3, T$_3$**   triiodothyronine.

**T4, T$_4$**   thyroxine.

**tab.**   tablet.

**TB**   tuberculosis.

**TBI**   **1.** traumatic brain injury. **2.** total body irradiation.

**Tbsp, tbsp.**   tablespoon; tablespoons.

**TBV**   total blood volume.

**TCA**   tricyclic antidepressant.

**TCM**   traditional Chinese medicine.

**TDD**   telecommunications device for the deaf.

**TDM**   therapeutic drug monitoring.

**temp, temp.** /tĕmp/   temperature.

**TENS** /tĕnz/   transcutaneous electrical nerve stimulation.

**THC**   tetrahydrocannabinol.

**Thr**   threonine.

**THR**   **1.** target heart rate. **2.** threshold heart rate. **3.** total hip replacement. **4.** thyroid hormone receptor.

**Ti**   titanium.

**TIA**   transient ischemic attack.

**tid, t.i.d.**   three times a day, used in writing prescriptions.

**TL**   thallium

**TLC**   total lung capacity.

**TMJ**   temporomandibular joint.

**TNF**   tumor necrosis factor.

**TNM**   tumor-node-metastasis.

**tPA, TPA**   tissue plasminogen activator.

**TPN**   total parenteral nutrition.

**TPR**   temperature, pulse, respiration.

**Trp**   tryptophan.

**TSE**   1. transmissible spongiform encephalopathy, any of a group of brain diseases, such as kuru or Creutzfeldt-Jakob's disease, in which the brain matter deteriorates. *See also* spongiform encephalopathy. 2. testicular self-examination.
**TSH**   thyroid-stimulating hormone.
**tsp.**   teaspoon; teaspoons.
**TSS**   toxic shock syndrome.
**TTP**   thrombotic thrombocytopenic purpura.
**TUR**   transurethral resection.
**TURP** /tûrp/   transurethral resection of the prostate.

**u**   atomic mass unit.
**U**   1. uranium. 2. unit; units. 3. uracil. 4. urine.
**UA, U/A**   urinalysis.
**UBT**   urea breath test.
**UGI**   upper gastrointestinal.
**ung, ung.**   ointment.
**UNOS** /yo͞o′nŏs/   United Network for Organ Sharing.
**UR**   ultraviolet radiation.
**URI**   upper respiratory infection.
**URTI**   upper respiratory tract infection.
**USDA**   United States Department of Agriculture (www.usda.gov).
**USFDA**   United States Food and Drug Administration (www.fda.gov).
**USP**   *United States Pharmacopeia.*
**USP-NF**   *United States Pharmacopeia—National Formulary.*
**UTI**   urinary tract infection.
**UV**   ultraviolet.
**UV**   radiation ultraviolet radiation.

**VA**   1. vertebral artery. 2. Veterans Administration 3. visual acuity. 4. volt-ampere.
**VAD**   1. vascular access device. 2. vascular assist device; ventricular assist device.
**Val**   valine.
**VATS**   video-assisted thoracoscopy.
**VC**   1. vital capacity. 2. vocal cord; vocal cords.
**VCU**   voiding cystourethrography.
**VCUG**   voiding cystourethrogram/cystourethrography.
**VD**   venereal disease.
**VF**   1. visual field. 2. ventricular fibrillation.
**Vfib** /vē′fĭb′/   ventricular fibriilation.
**VHDL**   very-high-density lipoprotein.
**VLDL**   very-low-density lipoprotein.
**V/Q**   ventilation-perfusion.
**VS**   vital sign; vital signs.
**VT**   ventricular tachycardia.
**V-tach** /vē′tăk′/   ventricular tachycardia.
**VSD**   ventricular septal defect.

**WAIS**   Wechsler Adult Intelligence Scale.
**WBC**   1. white blood cell. 2. white blood (cell) count.
**WBC count**   white blood cell count.
**WBC differential** /dĭf′ə rĕn′shəl/   white blood cell differential.
**WC**   wheelchair.
**WHO**   World Health Organization (www.who.int).
**WlSC** /wĭsk/   Wechsler Intelligence Scale for Children.
**wt, wt.**   weight.

**XRT**   radiation therapy.

**ZIFT**   zygote intrafallopian transfer.

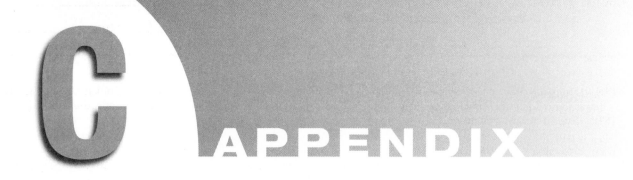

# Laboratory Testing and Normal Reference Values

Health care professional order laboratory tests to diagnose diseases, conditions, and to assess the general health and functioning of various parts of the body. The basic types of tests are blood tests, urinalysis, stool tests, and spinal taps, which analyze spinal fluid to look for diseases, such as meningitis.

## Blood Tests

The two most common blood tests are the complete blood count (CBC) and the blood culture. The CBC measures levels of substances in the blood as described in the following paragraphs. The blood culture is a test for bacteria or yeast. Blood is cultured in the laboratory and is bacteria or yeast is present, it is analyzed for what type it is and what infection it indicates.

### The CBC

The CBC tests for electrolytes by measuring levels of sodium, potassium, chloride, and bicarbonate in the body. It also measures other substances, such as blood urea, nitrogen, glucose, and sugars. In addition, it measures the red blood cells, white blood cells, and platelets to look for signs of anemia or infection.

**Sodium** plays a major role in regulating the amount of water in the body. Also, sodium is necessary for many body functions, like transmitting electrical signals in the brain. The test determines whether there's the right balance of sodium and liquid in the blood to carry out important bodily functions. High levels of sodium can lead to certain conditions, such as high blood pressure.

**Potassium** is essential to regulate how the heart beats. When potassium levels are too high or too low, it can increase the risk of an abnormal heartbeat. Low potassium levels are also associated with muscle weakness.

**Chloride** also helps maintain a balance of fluids in the body.

**Bicarbonate** prevents the body's tissues from getting too much or too little acid. The kidney and lungs balance the levels of bicarbonate in the body. So if bicarbonate levels are abnormal, it might indicate that there is a problem with those organs.

**Blood urea nitrogen (BUN)** is a measure of how well the kidneys are working.

**Creatinine** levels in the blood that are too high can indicate that the kidneys aren't working properly. The kidneys filter and excrete creatinine. Both dehydration and muscle damage also can raise creatinine levels.

**Glucose** is the main type of sugar in the blood. Glucose levels that are too high or too low can cause problems and are often caused by diabetes.

Three tests that are part of a CBC measure red blood cell (RBC) count, hemoglobin, and mean (red) cell volume (MCV). These test anemia, a common condition that occurs when there aren't enough red blood cells.

- The red blood cell count is a measure of the number of RBCs in the body.
- Hemoglobin is the oxygen-carrying protein in red blood cells. RBCs carry oxygen to all parts of the body.
- MCV measures the average size of the red blood cells.

Other tests include the **hematocrit** (HCT), which is the percentage of red blood cells in the blood sample. This is also a test for anemia.

**Also part of the CBC is the blood differential test that measures the relative numbers of white blood cells (WBCs) in the blood. WBCs (also called leukocytes) help the body fight infection. An abnormal white blood cell count may indicate that there is an infection, inflammation, or other stress in the body. There are five types of white blood cells: neutrophils, lymphocytes, eosinophils, basophils, and monocytes.**

Platelets are the smallest blood cells and are important to blood clotting and the prevention of excessive bleeding. If the platelet count is too low, a person can be in danger of bleeding in any part of the body.

## Blood Cultures

Blood is cultured when an infection or the condition of sepsis is suspected. Bacteria or yeast will show up in the blood culture if such conditions exist. Blood cultures are usually done twice if there is a positive result since false positives can lead to unnecessary treatment.

## Urinalysis

The kidneys make urine as they filter wastes from the bloodstream while leaving substances in the blood that the body needs, like protein and glucose. Urinalysis checks for the presence of protein and glucose in the urine as well as other substances that can indicate infection, poor function of a body part, or the presence of illegal drugs. The urine is checked for blood as well as many other substances and is an important diagnostic tool.

## Stool Test

The most common reason to collect stool is to determine whether a type of bacteria or parasite may be infecting the intestine. Stool is also checked for occult blood, possibly indicative of internal bleeding. Stool samples are also sometimes analyzed for the substances they contain. Some substances may indicated digestive disorders.

## Spinal Tap

A spinal tap or lumbar puncture (LP) is a procedure in which a small amount of the fluid that surrounds the brain and spinal cord, called the cerebrospinal fluid (CSF), is removed and examined. The fluid is examined for meningitis and other diseases of the central nervous system.

## Tests

The table that follows lists many of the laboratory tests that you will encounter in your allied health career. The table gives the normal ranges expected for each test.

## Table of laboratory tests

The table below lists a number of common laboratory tests taken either in normal CBCs (complete blood counts) or a urinalysis or as separate diagnostic tools.

Abbreviations used in table:

| | | | |
|---|---|---|---|
| W | women | mol | mole |
| M | men | l | liter |
| d | deci | m | milli |
| g | gram | m | micro |
| k | kilo | n | nano |
| kat | katal (unit of catalytic activity) | p | pico |

Note that "normal" values can vary depending on a variety of factors, including the patient's age or gender, time of day test was taken, and so on. In addition, as new medical advances are made, the understanding of what is the best range for some readings has changed. For example, optimal blood pressure readings are now lower than they were ten years ago.

| Laboratory Test | Normal Range in US Units | Normal Range in SI Units | To Convert US to SI Units |
|---|---|---|---|
| ALT (Alanine *aminotransferase) | W 7-30 units/liter M 10-55 units/liter | W 0.12-0.50 mkat/liter M 0.17-0.92 mkat/liter | x 0.01667 |
| Albumin | 3.1–4.3 g/dl | 31–43 g/liter | x 10 |
| Alkaline Phosphatase | W 30-100 units/liter M 45-115 units/liter | W 0.5-1.67 mkat/liter M 0.75-1.92 mkat/liter | x 0.01667 |
| Aspartate aminotransferase | W 9-25 units/liter M 10-40 units/liter | W 0.15-0.42 mkat/liter M 0.17-0.67 mkat/liter | x 0.01667 |
| Basophils | 0-3% of lymphocytes | 0.0-0.3 fraction of white blood cells | x 0.01 |
| Bilirubin – Direct | 0.0-0.4 mg/dl | 0-7 mmol/liter | x 17.1 |
| Bilirubin – Total | 0.0-1.0 mg/dl | 0-17 mmol/liter | x 17.1 |
| Blood pressure | 120/80 millimeters of mercury (mmHg). Top number is systolic pressure, when heart is pumping. Bottom number is diastolic pressure when heart is at rest. Blood pressure can be too low (hypotension) or too high (hypertension). | | No conversion |
| Cholesterol, total Desirable Marginal High | <200 mg/dL 200–239 mg/dL >239 mg/dL | <5.17 mmol/liter 5.17–6.18 mmol/liter >6.18 mmol/liter | x 0.02586 |

*variant of transaminase.

| Laboratory Test | Normal Range in US Units | Normal Range in SI Units | To Convert US to SI Units |
|---|---|---|---|
| Cholesterol, LDL<br>Desirable<br>Marginal<br>High<br>Very high | <100 mg/dL<br>100–159 mg/dL<br>160–189 mg/dL<br>>190 mg/dL | <2.59 mmol/liter<br>2.59–4.14 mmol/liter<br>4.14–4.89 mmol/liter<br>>4.91 mmol/liter | x 0.02586 |
| Cholesterol, HDL<br>Desirable<br>Moderate<br>Low (heart risk) | >60 mg/dL<br>40-60 mg/dL<br><40 mg/dL | >1.55 mmol/liter<br>1.03–1.55 mmol/liter<br><1.03 mmol/liter | x 0.02586 |
| Eosinophils | 0-8% of white blood cells | 0.0–0.8 fraction of white blood cells | x 0.01 |
| Erythrocytes RBC | 4.0–6.0 ml (females slightly lower than males) | 4.0–6.0 $10^{12}$/liter | |
| Glucose, urine | <0.05 g/dl | <0.003 mmol/liter | x 0.05551 |
| Glucose, plasma °fasting reading— often in self-test | 70–110 mg/dl (nonfasting not to exceed 140 mg/dl) | 3.9–6.1 mmol/liter | x 0.05551 |
| Hematocrit | W 36.0%–46.0% of red blood cells<br>M 37.0%–49.0% of red blood cells | W 0.36–0.46 fraction of red blood cells<br>M 0.37–0.49 fraction of red blood cells | x 0.01 |
| Hemoglobin | W 12.0–16.0 g/dl<br>M 13.0–18.0 g/dl | W 7.4–9.9 mmol/liter<br>M 8.1–11.2 mmol/liter | x 0.6206 |
| Leukocytes (WBC) | 4.5–11.0x$10^3$/mm$^3$ | 4.5–11.0x$10^9$/liter | x $10^6$ |
| Lymphocytes | 16%–46% of white blood cells | 0.16–0.46 fraction of white blood cells | x 0.01 |
| Mean corpuscular hemoglobin (MCH) | 25.0–35.0 pg/cell | 25.0–35.0 pg/cell | No conversion |
| Mean corpuscular hemoglobin concentration (MCHC) | 31.0–37.0 g/dl | 310–370 g/liter | x 10 |
| Mean corpuscular volume (MCV) | W 78–102 mm$^3$<br>M 78–100 mm$^3$<br>M 78–100 fl | W 78–102 fl | No conversion |
| Monocytes | 4–11% of white blood cells | 0.04–0.11 fraction of white blood cells | x 0.01 |
| Neutrophils | 45%–75% of white blood cells | 0.45–0.75 fraction of white blood cells | x 0.01 |

(*Continued*)

| Laboratory Test | Normal Range in US Units | Normal Range in SI Units | To Convert US to SI Units |
|---|---|---|---|
| Potassium | 3.4–5.0 mmol/liter | 3.4–5.0 mmol/liter | No conversion |
| Prostate specific antigen (PSA) | 0–2.5 ng/ml | | |
| Serum calcium | 8.5–10.5 mg/dl | 2.1–2.6 mmol/liter | x 0.25 |
| Sodium | 135–145 mmol/liter | 135–145 mmol/liter | No conversion |
| Testosterone, total (morning sample) | W 6–86 ng/dl<br>M 270-1070 ng/dl | W 0.21–2.98 nmol/liter<br>M 9.36-37.10 nmol/liter | x 0.03467 |
| Testosterone, unbound<br>Age 20–40<br><br>Age 41–60<br><br>Age 61–80 | W 0.6–3.1,<br>M 15.0–40.0 pg/ml<br>W 0.4–2.5,<br>M 13.0–35.0 pg/ml<br>W 0.2–2.0,<br>M 12.0–28.0 pg/ml | W 20.8–107.5,<br>M 520–1387 pmol/liter<br>W 13.9–86.7,<br>M 451–1213 pmol/liter<br>W 6.9–69.3,<br>M 416–971 pmol/liter | x 34.67 |
| Triglycerides, fasting<br>Normal<br>Borderline<br>High<br>Very high | 40–150 mg/dl<br>150–200 mg/dl<br>200–500 mg/dl<br>>500 mg/dl | 0.45–1.69 mmol/liter<br>1.69–2.26 mmol/liter<br>2.26–-5.65 mmol/liter<br>>5.65 mmol/liter | x 0.01129 |
| Urea, plasma (BUN)<br>Urinalysis pH | 8–25 mg/dl<br>5.0–9.0 | 2.9–8.9 mmol/liter<br>5.0–9.0 | x 0.357<br>No conversion |
| Specific gravity | 1.001–1.035 | 1.001–1.035 | |
| WBC (White blood cells, leukocytes) | $4.5–11.0 \times 10^3/mm^3$ | $4.5–11.0 \times 10^9$ liter | $x\ 10^6$ |

Table adapted from www.aidsinfonet.org

# APPENDIX D

# Complementary and Alternative Medicine (CAM)

The National Institutes of Health has established a department dealing with complementary and alternative medicine (NCCAM). The following information is from the NIH website (www.nih.gov) and gives an overview of complementary and alternative medicine practices that are currently being studied by NCCAM.

## What is CAM?

- Complementary medicine is used **together with** conventional medicine. An example of a complementary therapy is using aromatherapy to help lessen a patient's discomfort following surgery.
- Alternative medicine is used **in place of** conventional medicine. An example of an alternative therapy is using a special diet to treat cancer instead of undergoing surgery, radiation, or chemotherapy that has been recommended by a conventional doctor.

## Major Types of Complementary and Alternative Medicine?

NCCAM classifies CAM therapies into five categories, or domains:

## 1. Alternative Medical Systems

Alternative medical systems are built upon complete systems of theory and practice. Often, these systems have evolved apart from and earlier than the conventional medical approach used in the United States. Examples of alternative medical systems that have developed in Western cultures include homeopathic medicine and naturopathic medicine. Examples of systems that have developed in non-Western cultures include traditional Chinese medicine and Ayurveda. Some of the alternative systems are discussed in detail below.

### Traditional Chinese Medicine

TCM is a complete system of healing that dates back to 200 B.C. in written form. Korea, Japan, and Vietnam have all developed their own unique versions of traditional medicine based on practices originating in China. In the TCM view, the body is a delicate balance of two opposing and inseparable forces: yin and yang. Yin represents the cold, slow, or passive principle, while yang represents the hot, excited, or active principle. Among the major assumptions in TCM are that health is achieved by maintaining the body in a "balanced state" and that disease is due to an internal imbalance of yin and yang. This imbalance leads to blockage in the flow of qi (or vital energy) and of blood along pathways known as meridians. TCM practitioners typically use herbs, acupuncture, and massage to help unblock qi and blood in patients in an attempt to bring the body back into harmony and wellness.

Treatments in TCM are typically tailored to the subtle patterns of disharmony in each patient and are based on an individualized diagnosis. The diagnostic tools differ from those of conventional medicine. There are three main therapeutic modalities:

1. Acupuncture and moxibustion (moxibustion is the application of heat from the burning of the herb moxa at the acupuncture point)
2. Chinese Materia Medica (the catalogue of natural products used in TCM)
3. Massage and manipulation

Although TCM proposes that natural products catalogued in Chinese Materia Medica or acupuncture can be used alone to treat virtually any illness, quite often they are used together and sometimes in combination with other modalities (e.g., massage, moxibustion, diet changes, or exercise).

## Ayurvedic Medicine

Ayurveda, which literally means "the science of life," is a natural healing system developed in India. Ayurvedic texts claim that the sages who developed India's original systems of meditation and yoga developed the foundations of this medical system. It is a comprehensive system of medicine that places equal emphasis on the body, mind, and spirit, and strives to restore the innate harmony of the individual. Some of the primary Ayurvedic treatments include diet, exercise, meditation, herbs, massage, exposure to sunlight, and controlled breathing. In India, Ayurvedic treatments have been developed for various diseases (e.g., diabetes, cardiovascular conditions, and neurological disorders). However, a survey of the Indian medical literature indicates that the quality of the published clinical trials generally falls short of contemporary methodological standards with regard to criteria for randomization, sample size, and adequate controls.

## Naturopathy

Naturopathy is a system of healing, originating from Europe, that views disease as a manifestation of alterations in the processes by which the body naturally heals itself. It emphasizes health restoration as well as disease treatment. The term "naturopathy" literally translates as "nature disease." Today naturopathy, or naturopathic medicine, is practiced throughout Europe, Australia, New Zealand, Canada, and the United States. There are six principles that form the basis of naturopathic practice in North America (not all are unique to naturopathy):

1. The healing power of nature
2. Identification and treatment of the cause of disease
3. The concept of "first do no harm"
4. The doctor as teacher
5. Treatment of the whole person
6. Prevention

The core modalities supporting these principles include diet modification and nutritional supplements, herbal medicine, acupuncture and Chinese medicine, hydrotherapy, massage and joint manipulation, and lifestyle counseling. Treatment protocols combine what the practitioner deems to be the most suitable therapies for the individual patient.

## Homeopathy

Homeopathy is a complete system of medical theory and practice. Its founder, German physician Samuel Christian Hahnemann (1755-1843), hypothesized that one can select therapies on the basis of how closely symptoms produced by a remedy match the symptoms of the patient's disease. He called this the "principle of similars." Hahnemann proceeded to give repeated doses of many common remedies to healthy volunteers and carefully record the symptoms they produced. This procedure is called a "proving" or, in modern homeopathy, a "human pathogenic trial." As a result of this experience, Hahnemann developed his treatments for sick patients by matching the symptoms produced by a drug to symptoms in sick patients. Hahnemann emphasized from the beginning that carefully examining all aspects of a person's health status, including emotional and mental states, and tiny idiosyncratic characteristics, was essential.

## 2.   Mind-Body Interventions

Mind-body medicine uses a variety of techniques designed to enhance the mind's capacity to affect bodily function and symptoms. Some techniques that were considered CAM in the past have become mainstream (for example, patient support groups and cognitive-behavioral therapy). Other mind-body techniques are still considered CAM, including meditation, prayer, mental healing, and therapies that use creative outlets such as art, music, or dance.

## 3.   Biologically Based Therapies

Biologically based therapies in CAM use substances found in nature, such as herbs, foods, and vitamins. Some examples include dietary supplements, herbal products, and the use of other so-called natural but as yet scientifically unproven therapies (for example, using shark cartilage to treat cancer).

NCCAM lists herbs and supplements and their uses on their website. Many of these herbs have been used for centuries but have not necessarily been scientifically tested. It is important to note that herbs can be powerful supplements and can have allergic and drug interactions that may be serious. On the other hand, many people have found herbal remedies very useful. The following table lists some of the herbs currently recognized by NCCAM and, in many cases, under study for effectiveness. This table does not include vitamin supplements which have current established guidelines for daily intake.

| Herb | Where Found | Potential Uses |
| --- | --- | --- |
| alfalfa | legume crop widely grown | lowering of blood cholesterol and glucose |
| aloe vera | gel found in leaves of aloe vera plants | topical use in dermatology for wounds, skin infections, burns, etc. |
| astragalus | Chinese herb | used to treat many major illnesses in Traditional Chinese Medicine, such as cancer, heart disease, infections, and so on |
| barley | widely grown grain crop | lowering cholesterol, high fiber |
| belladonna | widely available | long used for pain and inflammation, such as headache, menstrual symptoms, etc. |
| beta-carotene | found in colorful fruits, grains, and vegetables | important antioxidant, essential to sight, bone development, and other bodily functions |

*(Continued)*

| Herb | Where Found | Potential Uses |
|---|---|---|
| bilberry | a berry closely related to blueberry | used to treat various inflammations |
| black cohosh | herb | treatment of hormonal difficulties, such as menopausal symptoms |
| black tea | shrubs grown in China and other parts of Asia | antioxidant, contains caffeine, a stimulant, acts as a diuretic |
| bromelain | extracted from the stem of pineapple plants | used to enhance digestion and as an anti-inflammatory |
| burdock | plant with fruits | used for various ailments, such as arthritis; fruit is sometimes used in treating diabetes. |
| calendula (marigold) | plant | wound-healing |
| chamomile | plant | widely used for sleep disorders, digestion, and many other conditions |
| clove | cultivated in Africa, Asia, and South America | topical antiseptic; anesthetic, and other uses |
| cranberry | berry grown mainly in North America | prevention of urinary tract infections; may be useful in treating other infections |
| dandelion | plant found wild in pastures and cultivated in certain areas | widely used for a variety of ailments; respiratory diseases; liver ailments; hepatitis; digestive disorders; and others |
| devil's claw | southern African plant | used to treat fever and malaria plus other conditions |
| dong quai | plant found widely in Asia | used to treat the female reproductive system in Traditional Chinese Medicine |
| echinacea | flowering plant | widely believed to have immune-enhancing properties |
| elder | tree | flowers, berries, and leaves are used in analgesics, as a diuretic, a laxative, and an emetic; also, an antioxidant |
| eucalyptus oil | plant | used as an anti-inflammatory agent, particularly in upper respiratory infections |
| evening primrose oil | oil extracted from herb | believed to improve diseases affected by essential fatty acids |

| Herb | Where Found | Potential Uses |
|------|-------------|----------------|
| feverfew | herb | anti-pyretic |
| flaxseed/flaxseed oil | widely grown plant | essential fatty acid; thought to be helpful in coronary artery disease |
| garlic | widely cultivated bulb | used to lower blood pressure, aid in gastric problems, and thought to have some anti-cancer properties |
| ginger | underground stems of plant | used widely in Asian medicine as a digestive agent; antitussive, and other uses |
| gingko | leaves of a tree | used for centuries in Asian medicine for a various of mental conditions, reduction of fatigue, and many other uses |
| ginseng | plant | used widely in Asian medicine and now worldwide for many conditions, including mental conditions, heart disease, immune disorders, and so on |
| goldenseal | herb | used for upper respiratory ailments, eardrops, and as part of laxatives, cleansers, and so on |
| green tea | leaves of the tea plant | antioxidant, stimulant |
| gymnema | herb | lowers blood glucose |
| hops | crop plant | relaxation and sedative effects |
| horse chestnut | seed extract from tree | used in chronic venous insufficiency |
| horsetail | herb | used to treat edema |
| kava | roots of a shrub | used to treat anxiety |
| lavender | herb | relaxation effects |
| licorice | roots of a shrub | used for upper respiratory ailments |
| milk thistle | plant | treatment of liver and gallbladder disorders |
| passion flower | flowering plant | used as a sedative and in digestive disorders |

*(Continued)*

| Herb | Where Found | Potential Uses |
|---|---|---|
| peppermint | flowering plant | widely used for upper respiratory, indigestion, joint pain, nausea, and many other uses |
| propolis | natural resin created by bees | used as an antiviral; used to reduce dental caries and as an anti-infective agent |
| psyllium | cultivated crop | high fiber plant used as a laxative |
| pygeum | bark of an African evergreen | used in bladder and urinary disorders |
| red clover | legume | used to treat menopausal symptoms and for asthma and pertussis |
| red yeast rice | product of yeast grown on rice | cholesterol-lowering agent |
| saw palmetto | plant | used to treat prostate conditions |
| seaweed; kelp | grown in coastal waters | widely used as a food and medicine for tumors, ulcers, headaches, digestive disorders, and many others |
| soy | cultivated food crop | used in some estrogen disorders |
| St. John's wort | flowering plant | antidepressant |
| tea tree oil | distilled from the leaves of a plant | used as a topical antifungal |
| turmeric | root of a plant | anti-inflammatory; antioxidant; digestive disorders, and other uses |
| valerian | herb | widely used for heart disease, UTIs, insomnia, angina, and other uses |
| white horehound | herb | expectorant |
| wild yam | plant | used to treat menopausal symptoms |
| yohimbe | bark of a tree | male impotence |

## 4.  Manipulative and Body-Based Methods

Manipulative and body-based methods in CAM are based on manipulation and/or movement of one or more parts of the body. Some examples include chiropractic or osteopathic manipulation, and massage. The following is a list of some specific manipulative and body-based methods.

- **Alexander technique:** Patient education/guidance in ways to improve posture and movement, and to use muscles efficiently.
- **Bowen technique:** Gentle massage of muscles and tendons over acupuncture and reflex points.
- **Chiropractic manipulation:** Adjustments of the joints of the spine, as well as other joints and muscles.
- **Craniosacral therapy:** Form of massage using gentle pressure on the plates of the patient's skull.
- **Feldenkrais method:** Group classes and hands-on lessons designed to improve the coordination of the whole person in comfortable, effective, and intelligent movement.
- **Massage therapy:** Assortment of techniques involving manipulation of the soft tissues of the body through pressure and movement.
- **Osteopathic manipulation:** Manipulation of the joints combined with physical therapy and instruction in proper posture.
- **Reflexology:** Method of foot (and sometimes hand) massage in which pressure is applied to "reflex" zones mapped out on the feet (or hands).
- **Rolfing:** Deep tissue massage (also called structural integration).
- **Trager bodywork:** Slight rocking and shaking of the patient's trunk and limbs in a rhythmic fashion.
- **Tui Na:** Application of pressure with the fingers and thumb, and manipulation of specific points on the body (acupoints).

## 5.  Energy Therapies

Energy therapies involve the use of energy fields. They are of two types:

- **Biofield therapies** are intended to affect energy fields that purportedly surround and penetrate the human body. The existence of such fields has not yet been scientifically proven. Some forms of energy therapy manipulate biofields by applying pressure and/or manipulating the body by placing the hands in, or through, these fields. Examples include qi gong, Reiki, and Therapeutic Touch.
- **Bioelectromagnetic-based therapies** involve the unconventional use of electromagnetic fields, such as pulsed fields, magnetic fields, or alternating-current or direct-current fields.

# E APPENDIX

# Selected List of English-Spanish Medical Terms

The following list gives Spanish translations for some common medical terms. In your allied health career, you are likely to come in contact with patients who are primarily Spanish-speaking. This appendix is a valuable reference tool for such situations.

**abortifacient** (abortifaciente)
**abortion** (aborto)
**abscess** (absceso)
**absorption** (absorción)
**acetabulum** (acetábulo)
**acetone** (acetona)
**acetylcholine** (acetilcolina)
**achalasia** (acalasia)
**acidosis** (acidosis)
**acne** (acne)
**acne vulgaris** (acné vulgar)
**acromegaly** (acromegalia)
**acromion** (acromion)
**Adam's apple** (manzana de adán)
**adenoidectomy** (adenoidectomía)
**adenoiditis** (adenoiditis)
**adenoids** (adenoides)
**adipose** (adiposo)
**adrenal** (adrenal)
**adrenalectomy** (adrenalectomía)
**adrenaline** (adrenalina)
**afterbirth** (secundina)
**agglutination** (aglutinación)
**agglutinogen** (aglutinógeno)
**agnosia** (agnosia)
**agranulocyte** (agranulocito)
**albinism** (albinismo)
**albumin** (albúmina)
**albuminuria** (albuminuria)
**aldosterone** (aldosterina)
**allergen** (alergeno)
**allergy** (alergia)
**allograft** (aloinjerto)
**alopecia** (alopecia)
**alopecia areata** (alopecia areata)
**alveolus, pl. alveoli** (alvéolo)
**amenorrhea** (amenorrea)
**amino acid, AA** (aminoácido(AA))
**amnesia** (amnesia)

**amniocentesis** (amniocentesis)
**amnios** (amnion)
**amniotic** (aminiótico)
**amphiarthroses** (anfiartroses)
**amputation** (amputación)
**amylase** (amilasa)
**anacusis** (anacusia)
**analgesic** (analgésico)
**anaphylaxis** (anafilaxia o anafilaxis)
**anastomosis** (anastomosis)
**androgen** (andrógeno)
**anemia** (anemia)
**anesthetic** (anestésico)
**aneurysm** (aneurisma)
**angina** (angina)
**angina pectoris** (angina de pecho)
**angioplasty** (angioplastia)
**angioscopy** (angioscopia)
**anisocytosis** (anisocitosis)
**ankle** (tobillo)
**ankyloglossia** (anquiloglosia)
**ankylosis** (anquilosis)
**anorchism, anorchia** (anorquia)
**anthracosis** (antracosis)
**antibacterial** (antibacteriano)
**antibiotic** (antibiótico)
**antibody** (anticuerpo)
**antidiabetic** (antidiabético)
**antidote** (antidoto)
**antifungal** (antifúngico)
**antigen** (antígeno)
**antihistamines** (antihistamines)
**antitoxin** (antitoxina)
**anuria** (anuria)
**anus** (ano)
**aorta** (aorta)
**apex** (apex)
**aphagia** (afagia)
**aphakia** (afaquia)

aphasia (afasia)
apnea (apnea)
appendix (apéndice)
apraxia (apraxia)
arachnoid (aracnoideo)
areola (aréola)
arrhythmia (arritmia)
arteriole (arteriola)
arteriosclerosis (arteriosclerosis)
arteritis (arteritis)
artery (arteria)
arthralgia (artralgia)
arthritis (artritis)
arthrocentesis (artrocentesis)
articulation (articulación)
asbestosis (asbestosis)
ascites (ascitis)
aspermia (aspermia)
aspiration (aspiración)
asthenopia (astenopía)
asthma (asma)
astigmatism (astimagtismo)
astrocyte, astroglia (astrocito, astroglia)
astrocytoma (astrocitoma)
asystole (asistolia)
ataxia (ataxia)
atelectasis (atelectasia)
atheroma (ateroma)
atherosclerosis (ateriosclerosis)
atlas (atlas)
atresia (atresia)
atrium, pl. atria (atrium, pl.atrio)
atrophy (atrofia)
audiogram (audiograma)
audiologist (audiólogo)
audiometry (audiometría)
aura (aura)
auricle (auricular)
auscultation (auscultatión)
autograft (autoinjerto)
axis (axis)
axon (axón)
Azoospermia (azoospermia)
azotemia (azoemia)

bacillus (bacillo)
balanitis (balanitis)
base (base)
basophil (basófilo)
basophilia (basofilia)
bile (bilis)
bilirubin (bilirrubina)
biopsy (biopsia)
blackhead (punto negro)
bladder (vejiga)
blepharitis (blefaritis)

blindness (ceguera)
blood (sangre)
body (cuerpo)
bone (hueso)
brachytherapy (braquiterapia)
bradycardia (bradicardia)
bradypnea (bradipnea)
brain (cerebro)
brainstem (tronco encefálico)
bronchiole (bronquiolo)
bronchitis (bronquitis)
bronchodilators (broncodilatador)
bronchography (broncografía)
bronchoplasty (broncoplastia)
bronchoscope (broncoscopio)
bronchus, pl. bronchi (bronquio)
bronchospasm (broncoespasmo)
bruit (ruido)
bulla (pl. bullae) (bulla)
bunion (bunio)
bunionectomy (bunionectomía)
burn (quemadura)
bursa pl. bursae (bursa)
bursa, pl. bursae (bolso)
bursectomy (bursectomía)
bursitis (bursitis)

calcaneus (calcáneo)
calcar (calcar)
calcitonin (calcitona)
calcium (calico)
callus (callo)
cancellous (canceloso)
candidiasis (candidiasis)
capillary (capilar)
carbon dioxide (dióxido de carbono)
carbuncle (carbunco)
cardiomyopathy (cardiomiopatía)
cartilage (cartílago)
casting (colado)
castration (castración)
cataract (catarata)
catecholamines (catecolaminas)
cauterization (cauterización)
cauterize (cauterizar)
cecum (ciego)
cellulitis (celulitis)
cerebellitis (cerebelitis)
cerebrum (cerebrum)
cervix (cervix)
chalazion (chalazión)
cheeks (carrillo)
cheilitis (queilitis)
chemotherapy (quimioterapia)
chlamydia (clamidia)
chloasma (cloasma)

cholangitis (colangitis)
cholecystectomy (colecistectomía)
cholecystitis (colecistitis)
cholecystography (colecistografía)
cholesterol (colesterol)
chondromalacia (condromalacia)
chorion (corion)
choroid (coroides)
chyme (quimo)
cicatrix, scar (cicatriz)
circumsicion (circumcisión)
cirrhosis (cirrosis)
claudication (claudicación)
clavicle (clavícula)
climacteric (climaterio)
clitoris (clíctoris)
coagulation (coagulación)
coccyx (cóccix)
cochlea (caracol)
coitus (coito)
colectomy (colectomía)
colic (cólico)
colitis (colitis)
collagen (colágeno)
colon (colon)
colonoscopy (colonoscopia)
colostomy (colostomía)
coma (coma)
concussion (concusión)
condom (condón)
conductivity (conductividad)
condyloma (condiloma)
cones (conos)
conization (conización)
conjunctivitis (conjunctivitis)
conjuntiva, pl. conjunctivae (conjuntiva)
constipation (constipación)
constriction (constricción)
contraception (anticoncepción)
convolution (circunvolución)
copulation (copulación)
cordotomy (cordotomía)
corium (corium)
corn (callo)
cornea (cornea)
cortex (corteza)
corticosteroid (cortico teroide)
cortisol (cortisol)
craniectomy (craniet  ía)
craniotomy (craneoto  ía)
creatine (creatina)
creatinine (creatinina
crest (cresta)
croup (crup)
crust (costar)
cryosurgery (criocirugía)
cuticle (cutícula)

cyanosis (cianosis)
cystectomy (cistectomía)
cystitis (cistitis)
cystocele (cistocele)
cystolith (cistolito)
cystorrhaphy (cistorrafia)
cystoscopy (cistoscopia)

deafness (sordera)
decibel (decibel)
decubitus (decúbito)
defecation (defecación)
deglutition (deglución)
dementia (demencia)
dendrite (dentrita)
depolarization (despolarización)
dermabrasion (dermabrasión)
dermatitis (dermatitis)
dermatochalasis (dermatocalasia)
dermatology (dermatología)
dermis (dermis)
desmielinación (demyelination)
diabetes (diabetes)
diaphoresis (diaforesis)
diaphragm (diaphragma)
diaphysis (diáfisis)
diarrhea (diarrhea)
diastole (diástole)
diencephalon (diencéfalo)
digestion (digestion)
diphtheria (difteria)
diplopia (diplopía)
disk, disc (disco)
diskography (discografía)
dislocation (dislocación)
diverticulitis (diverticulitis)
diverticulosis (diverticulosis)
dopamine (dopamina)
drug (droga)
druggist (boticario)
duodenum (duodeno)
dwarfism (enanismo)
dyscrasia (discrasia)
dysentery (disentería)
dysmenorrhea (dismenorrea)
dyspareunia (disparfor unia)
dyspepsia (dispepsia)
dysphagia (disfagia)
dysphasia (disfasia)
dysphonia (disfonía)
dyspnea (disnea)
dysrhythmia (disritmia)
dystonia (distonía)
dysuria (disuria)

ear (oreja, oído)
eardrum (tambor de oído)

**ecchymosis** (equimosis)
**echocardiographya** (ecocardiografía)
**eczema** (eccema)
**edema** (edema)
**ejaculation** (eyaculación)
**elbow** (codo)
**electroencephalograph** (electroencefalógrafo)
**electrolyte** (electrólito)
**electromyogram** (electromiógrafo)
**electrophoresis** (electroforesis)
**embolectomy** (embolectomía)
**embolus** (émbolo)
**emesis** (emesis)
**emphysema** (enfisema pulmonar)
**empyema** (empiema)
**encephalitis** (encefalitis)
**encephalogram** (encefalograma)
**endocarditis** (endocarditis)
**endocardium** (endocardio)
**endocrine gland** (glándula endocrina)
**endolymph** (endolinfa)
**endometriosis** (endometriosis)
**endometrium** (endometrio)
**endoscope** (endoscopio)
**endosteum** (endostio)
**endothelium** (endotelio)
**enteritis** (enteritis)
**enucleation** (enucleación)
**enuresis** (enuresis)
**enzyme** (enzima)
**eosinophil** (eosinófilo)
**eosinophilia** (eosinofilia)
**epicardium** (epicardio)
**epidermis** (epidermis)
**epididymis** (epidídimo)
**epididymitis** (epididimitis)
**epiglottis** (epiglotis)
**epinephrine** (epinefrina)
**epiphora** (epífora)
**epiphysitis** (epifisitis)
**epispadias** (epispadias)
**epithalamus** (epitálamo)
**equilibrium** (equilibrio)
**erosion** (erosion)
**eructation** (eructación)
**erythrocyte** (eritrocito)
**erythropenia** (eritropenia)
**erythropoietin** (eritropoyetina)
**esophagitis** (esofagitis)
**esophagoplasty** (esofagoplastia)
**esophagoscopy** (esofagoscopia)
**esophagus** (esófago)
**esotropia** (esotropía)
**estrogen** (estrógeno)
**eupnea** (eupnea)
**euthanasia** (euthanasia)
**excitability** (excitabilidad)

**excoriation** (excoriación)
**exhalation** (exahalación)
**exocrine** (exocrine)
**exocrine gland** (glándula ecrina)
**exophthalmos, exophthalmus** (exoftalmía)
**exostosis** (exostosis)
**expiration** (espiración)
**exudate** (exudado)
**eye** (ojo)
**eyebrow** (ceja)
**eyelashes** (pestaña)
**eyelid** (párpado)
**eyestrain** (vista fatigada)

**fascia** (fascia)
**feces** (heces)
**femur** (fémur)
**fibrillation** (fibrilación)
**fibrinogen** (fibrinógeno)
**fibroid** (fibroide)
**fibula** (peroné)
**filtration** (filtración)
**fimbriae** (fimbria)
**fissure** (fisura)
**flaccid** (flácido)
**flagellum** (flagelo)
**flatulence** (flatulencia)
**flatus** (flato)
**flutter** (aleteo)
**fontanelle** (fontanela)
**foramen magnum** (foramen magnum)
**foramen** (agujero)
**foreskin** (prepucio)
**fossa** (fosa)
**phosphorus** (fósforo)
**fracture** (fractura)
**frenulum** (frenillo)
**fulguration** (fulguración)
**fundus** (fondo)
**furuncle** (furúnculo)

**gait** (marcha)
**gallbladder** (vesícula biliar)
**gallop** (galope)
**gallstone** (cálculo biliar)
**gamete** (gameto)
**gangliitis** (ganglitis)
**ganglion** (ganglio)
**gangrene** (gangrena)
**gastrectomy** (gastrectomía)
**gastritis** (gastritis)
**gastroenteritis** (gastroenteritis)
**gastroscopy** (gastrocopia)
**generic** (genérico)
**genetics** (genética)
**gestation** (gestación)
**gigantism** (gigantismo)

**gland** (glándula)
**glaucoma** (glaucoma)
**glioma** (glioma)
**globin** (globina)
**globulin** (globulina)
**glomerulus, pl. glomuleri** (glomérulo)
**glossitis** (glositis)
**glottis** (glotis)
**glucagon** (glucagon)
**glucose** (glucosa)
**glycogen** (glucógeno)
**goiter** (bocio)
**gonad** (gónada)
**goniometer** (goniómetro)
**gonorrhea** (gonorrea)
**granulocytosis** (granulocitosis)
**gravida** (grávida)
**gum** (encía)
**gynecologist** (ginecólogo)

**hair root** (raíz de pelo)
**halitosis** (halitosis)
**hearing** (audición)
**heart** (corazón)
**heel** (talón)
**hematemesis** (hematemesis)
**hematocrit** (hematócrito)
**hematocytoblast** (hematocitoblasto)
**hematuria** (hematuria)
**hemodialysis** (hemodiálisis)
**hemoglobin** (hemoglobina)
**hemolysis** (hemólisis)
**hemophilia** (hemofilia)
**hemorrhoidectomy** (hemorroidectomía)
**hemorrhoids** (hemorroides)
**hemothorax** (hemotórax)
**heparin** (heparina)
**hepatitis** (hepatitis)
**hepatomegaly** (hepatomegalia)
**hepatopathy** (hepatopatía)
**hernia** (hernia)
**herniated disk** (disco herniated)
**herpes** (herpes)
**heterograft** (heteroinjerto)
**high blood pressure** (presión arterial alta)
**hilum, also hilus** (hilio)
**hirsutism** (hirsutimo)
**histamine** (histamine)
**histeroscopy** (histeroscopia)
**homograft** (homoinjerto)
**hordeolum** (orzuelo)
**hormone** (hormona)
**humerus** (húmero)
**hydrocephalus** (hidrocefalia)
**hymen** (himen)
**hyperopia** (hiperopía)

**hyperparathyroidism** (hiperparatiroidismo)
**hypersensitivity** (hipersensibilidad)
**hyperthyroidism** (hipertiroidism)
**hyperventilation** (hiperventilación)
**hypoadrenalism** (hipoadrenalismo)
**hypdermis** (hipodermis)
**hypoglycemia** (hipoglucemia)
**hypoglycemic** (hipoglucémico)
**hypoparathyroidism** (hipoparatiroidismo)
**hypopharynx** (hipofaringe)
**hypophysis** (hipófisis)
**hypospadias** (hiposoadias)
**hypotension** (hipotensión)
**hypothalamus** (hipotálamo)
**hypothyroidism** (hipotiroidismo)
**hypoventilation** (hipoventilación)
**hypoxemia** (hipoxemia)
**hypoxia** (hipoxia)
**hysterectomy** (histerectomía)
**hysterosalpingography** (histerosalpingografía)

**icterus** (icterus)
**ileitis** (ileitis):
**ileostomy** (ileostomía)
**ileum** (íleon)
**ileum** (ilium)
**ileus** (íleo)
**immunity** (inmunidad)
**immunoglobulin** (inmunoglobina)
**impetigo** (impetigo)
**impotence** (impotencia)
**incontinence** (incontinecia)
**incus** (incus)
**infarct, infarction** (infarto)
**infertility** (infertilidad)
**inhalation** (inhalación)
**insertion** (inserción)
**inspiration** (inspiración)
**insulin** (insulina)
**integument** (integumento)
**interleukin** (interleucina)
**interneuron** (interneuronas)
**intestine** (intestino)
**intradermal** (intradérmico)
**introitus** (introito)
**iridectomy** (iridectomía)
**iris** (iris)
**iritis** (iritis)
**ischemia** (isquemia)
**ischium** (isquión)
**isthmus** (istmo)
**IV** (intavenoso)

**jaundice** (ictericia)
**jejunum** (yeyuno)
**joint** (empalme)

keloid (queloide)
keratin (queratina)
keratitis (queratitis)
keratoplasty (queratoplastia)
keratosis (queratosis)
ketoacidosis (cetoacidosis)
ketone (cetona)
ketonuria (cetonuria)
ketosis (cetosis)
kidney (riñón)
kyphosis (cifosis)

lacrimation (lagrimeo)
lactation (lactación)
lactiferous (lactífero)
lamina, pl. laminae (lamina)
laparoscopy (laparoscopia)
laryngitis (laringitis)
laryngoplasty (laringoplastia)
laryngoscopy (laringoscopia)
laryngostomy (laringostomía)
larynx (laringe)
lens (lens)
lesion (lesión)
leukoderma (leucodermia)
leukoplakia (leucoplaquia)
leukorrhea (leucorrea)
ligament (ligamento)
lip (labio)
liver (hígado)
lobectomy (lobectomía)
lobotomy (lobotomía)
lordosis (lordosis)
low blood pressure (presión de arterial baja)
lumen (lumen)
lung (pulmón)
lunula (lúnula)
lymph (linfa)
lymphadenectomy (linfadenectomía)
lymphadenopathy (linfadenopatía)
lymphocyte (linfocito)
lymphoma (linfoma)

macrocytosis (macrocitosis)
macrophage (macrófago)
macule, macula (mácula)
malleus (malleus)
mammography (mamografía)
mammoplasty (mamoplastia)
mandible (mandíbula)
mastectomy (mastectomía)
mastication (masticación)
mastitis (mastitis)
meatus (meato)
mediastinum (mediastino)
medication, medicine (medicación)

medulla (médula)
megakaryocyte (megacariocito)
melanin (melanina)
melanocyte (melanocito)
melena (melena)
menarche (menarca)
meninges, sing. meninx (nenunges, sing. meningis)
meningioma (meningioma)
meningitis (meningitis)
meningocele (meningocele)
meningomyelocele (meningomielocele)
menopause (menopausia)
menorrhagia (menorragia)
menstruation (menstruación)
mesentery (mesenterio)
mesothelioma (mesotelioma)
metacarpal (metacarpiano)
metaphysic (metáfisis)
metastasis (metastasis)
metrorrhagia (metrorragia)
microcytosis (microcitosis)
microglia (microglia)
microphage (micrófago)
midbrain (cerebro medio)
miscarriage (aborto espontáneo)
monocyte (monocito)
mouth (boca)
murmur (soplo)
muscle (músculo)
muscular dystrophy (distrofia muscular)
musculoskeletal (musculoesquelético)
myalgia (mialgia)
myeloblast (mieloblasto)
myelogram (mielograma)
myelography (mielografía)
myeloma (mieloma)
myocarditis (miocarditis)
myocardium (miocardio)
myodynia (miodinia)
myoma (mioma)
myomectomy (miomectomía)
myometrium (miometrio)
myopia, nearsightedness (miopía)
myositis (miositis)
myringitis (miringitis)
myxedema (mixedema)

nail (uña)
narcolepsy (narcolepsia)
nasopharynx (nasofaringe)
nausea (nausea)
necrosis (necrosis)
neoplasm (neoplasma)
nephrectomy (nefrectomía)
nephritis (nefritis)
nephroblastoma (nefroblastoma)

**nerve** (nervio)
**neurectomy** (neurectomía)
**neurilemma** (neurilema)
**neuritis** (neuritis)
**neuron** (neurona)
**neurosurgeon** (neurocirujano)
**neurotransmitter** (neurotramisor)
**neutrophil** (neutrófilo)
**nevus** (nevo)
**nipple** (pezón)
**nocturia** (nocturia)
**lumpectomy** (nodulectomía)
**nodule** (nódulo)
**norepinephrine** (norepinefrina)
**nose** (nariz)
**nosebleed** (epistaxis)
**nostrils** (naris)
**NSAID** (agents de antiiflamatorios, AINE)
**nyctalopia** (nictalopía)
**nystagmus** (nistagmo)

**obesity** (obesidad)
**obstetrician** (obstetra)
**occlusion** (oclusión)
**olecranon** (olecranon)
**oligodendroglia** (oligodendroglia)
**oligodendroglioma** (oligodendroglioma)
**oligomenorrhea** (oligomenorrea)
**oligospermia** (oligospermia)
**oliguria** (oliguria)
**onychia, onychitis** (oniquia)
**onychopathy** (onicopatía)
**oocyte** (oocito)
**oophorectomy** (ooforectomía)
**ophthalmologist** (oftalmología)
**ophthalmoscopy** (oftalmoscópia)
**optometrist** (optometrista)
**orchidectomy** (orquidectomía)
**orchiectomy** (orquietomía)
**oropharynx** (orofaringe)
**orthopedist** (ortopedista)
**orthopnea** (ortopnea)
**orthosis, orthotics** (ortósis, ortótica)
**ossification** (osificación)
**ostealgia** (ostealgia)
**osteoarthritis** (osteoartritis)
**osteoblast** (osteoblasto)
**osteoclasis** (osteoclasia)
**osteoclast** (osteoclasto)
**osteocyte** (osteocito)
**osteodynia** (osteodinia)
**osteoma** (osteoma)
**osteomyelitis** (osteomielitis)
**osteopath** (osteópata)
**osteoplasty** (osteoplastia)
**osteoporosis** (osteoporosis)

**osteosarcoma** (osteosarcoma)
**osteotomy** (osteotomía)
**otalgia** (otalgia)
**otitis externa** (otitis externa)
**otitis media** (otitis media)
**otoliths** (otolito)
**otologist** (otólogo)
**otoplasty** (otoplastia)
**otorrhagia** (otorragia)
**otorrhea** (otorrea)
**otosclerosis** (otosclerosis)
**otoscopy** (otoscopia)
**ovary** (ovario)
**ovulation** (ovulación)
**ovum** (óvulo)
**oxytocin** (ositocina)
**oxytocin** (oxitocina)

**pacemaker** (marcapaso)
**palpitations** (palpitaciones)
**palsy** (parálisis)
**pancreas** (páncreas)
**pancreatectomy** (pancreatectomía)
**pancreatitis** (pancreatitis)
**pancytopenia** (pancitopenia)
**papilla** (papila)
**papule** (pápula)
**paracusis** (paracusia)
**paranychia** (paroniquia)
**parasiticide** (parasiticida)
**parathormone** (parathormona)
**parathyroid** (paratiroide)
**paroxysmal** (paroxístico)
**Parturition** (parturición)
**patella** (rótula)
**pathogen** (patógeno)
**pediculosis** (pediculosis)
**pelvis** (pelvis)
**pemphigus** (pénfigo)
**penis** (pene)
**pepsin** (pepsina)
**percussion** (percusión)
**pericarditis** (pericarditis)
**pericardium** (pericardio)
**perimetrium** (perimetrio)
**perineum** (perineo)
**periosteum** (periostio)
**peristalsis** (peristaltismo)
**peritoneoscopy** (peritoneoscopia)
**peritonitis** (peritonitis)
**pertussis** (pertussis)
**PET** (TEP)
**petechia** (petequia)
**phagocytosis** (fagocitosis)
**phalanges** (falange)
**pharmacology** (farmacología)

**pharyngitis** (faringitis)
**pharynx** (faringe)
**phimosis** (fimosis)
**phlebitis** (flebitis)
**phlebography** (flebografía)
**phlebotomy** (flebotomía)
**photophobia** (fotobia)
**pia mater** (piamadre)
**pinna** (pinna)
**placenta** (placenta)
**plaque, patch** (placa)
**plasma** (plasma)
**plasmapheresis** (plasmaféresis)
**platelet** (plaqueta)
**pleura, pl. pleurae** (pleura)
**pleuritis, pleurisy** (pleuritis)
**pneumoconiosis** (neumoconiosis)
**pneumonectomy** (neumonectomía)
**pneumonia** (neumonía)
**pneumonitis** (neumonitis)
**pneumothorax** (neumotórax)
**podagra** (podagra):
**podiatrist** (podiatra)
**poikilocytosis** (poiquilolocitosis)
**polarization** (polarización)
**polycythemia** (policetemia)
**polydipsia** (polidipsa)
**polyp** (pólipo)
**polypectomy** (polipectomía)
**polypoid** (polipoide)
**polyposis** (poliposis)
**polyuria** (poliuria)
**pons** (pons)
**pore** (poro)
**presbyacusis** (presbiacusia)
**presbyopia** (presbiopía)
**prescription** (perscripción)
**priapism** (priapismo)
**proctitis** (proctitis)
**proctoscopy** (proctoscopia)
**progesterone** (progesterona)
**prostate** (próstata)
**prostatectomy** (prostatectomía)
**prostatitis** (prostatitis)
**prothrombin** (protrombina)
**pruritus** (prurito)
**psoriasis** (psoriasis)
**puberty** (pubertad)
**pubes** (pubis)
**pulmonary artery** (arteria pulmunar)
**pulmonary valve** (válvula pulmonar)
**pulse** (pulso)
**pupil** (pupila)
**purpura** (púrpura)
**pustule** (pustule)
**pyelitis** (pielitis)

**pylorus** (píloro)
**pyoderma** (pioderma)
**pyuria** (piuria)

**radiculitis** (radiculitis)
**rales** (rales)
**receptor** (receptor)
**rectum** (recto)
**reduction** (reducción)
**reflejo** (reflex)
**reflux** (reflujo)
**refraction** (refracción)
**regurgitation** (regurgitación)
**renin** (renina)
**renogram** (renograma)
**repolarization** (repolarización)
**resectoscope** (resectoscopio)
**reticulocytosis** (reticulocitosis)
**retina** (retina)
**retinitis** (retinitis)
**retroflexion** (retroflexión)
**retroperitoneal** (retroperitoneal)
**retroversion** (retroversión)
**retrovirus** (retrovirus)
**rhabdomyoma** (rabdomioma)
**rhabdomyosarcoma** (rabdomiosarcoma)
**rheumatologist** (reumatologo)
**rhinitis** (rinitis)
**rhinoplasty** (rinoplastia)
**rhinorrhea** (rinorrea)
**rhonchi** (ronquido)
**rib** (costilla)
**rickets** (raquitismo)
**rigidity** (rigidez)
**rigor** (rigor)
**ringworm** (tiña)
**rods** (bastoncillos)
**roentgenology** (roentgenología)
**rosacea** (rosácea)
**rub** (roce)
**rubella, rubeola** (rubéola)
**rugae** (rugae)

**sacrum** (sacro)
**saliva** (saliva)
**salpingectomy** (salpingectomía)
**salpingitis** (salpingitis)
**sarcoidosis** (sarcoidosis)
**scabies** (sarna)
**scale** (costar)
**scale** (escala)
**scapula** (escápula)
**sciatica** (ciática)
**scirrhous** (escirroso)
**sclera** (esclerótica)
**scleritis** (escleritis)

**scleroderma** (esclerodermia)
**scoliosis** (escolisis)
**scotoma** (escotoma)
**scrotum** (escroto)
**seborrehea** (seborrhea)
**sebum** (sebo)
**sella turcica** (silla turcica)
**semen** (semen)
**septoplasty** (septoplastia)
**septostomy** (septostomía)
**pseudophakia** (seudofaquia)
**septum** (tabique)
**sequestrum** (secuetro)
**serum** (suero)
**shin** (espinilla)
**shingles** (culebrilla)
**sight** (vista)
**sigmoidoscopy** (sigmoidoscopia)
**singultus** (singulto)
**sinus** (seno)
**sinusitis** (sinusitis)
**skeleton** (esqueleto)
**skull** (cráneo)
**smell** (olfacción, oler)
**somnambulism** (sonambulismo)
**somnolence** (somnolencia)
**sonogram** (sonograma)
**sonography** (sonografía)
**spasm** (espasmo)
**sperm** (esperma)
**spermatozoon, pl. spermatozoa** (espermatozoo)
**spermicide** (espermicida)
**sphygmomanometer** (esfigmomanómetro)
**spina bifida** (espina bífida)
**spirometer** (espirómetro)
**spleen** (bazo)
**splenectomy** (esplenectomía)
**splinting** (ferulización)
**spondylolisthesis** (espondilolistesis)
**spondylolysis** (espodilólisis)
**spondylosyndesis** (espodilosindesis)
**sponge** (esponja)
**stapes, pl. stapes, stapedes** (estribo)
**steatorrhea** (esteatorrea)
**stenosis** (estenosis)
**sternum** (esternón)
**steroid** (steroide)
**stimulus** (estimulo)
**stomach** (estómago)
**strabismus** (estrabismo)
**stratum** (estrato)
**stratum corneum** (estrato córne)
**striae** (estría)
**stridor** (estridor)
**stroke** (accidente cerebrovascular)
**subluxation** (sublaxación)

**sulcus** (surco)
**suppository** (supositorio)
**suture** (sutura)
**sympathomimetic** (simpatomimético)
**symphysis** (sínfisis)
**synapse** (sinapsis)
**synarthrosis** (sinartrosis)
**syncope** (síncope)
**synovectomy** (sinovectomía)
**syphilis** (sífilis)
**syrine** (jeringa)
**labyrinthitis** (laberintitis)
**systole** (sístole)

**tachycardia** (taquicardia)
**tachypnea** (taquipnea)
**tears** (lágrimas)
**tendinitis, tendonitis** (tendonitis)
**tendon** (tendon)
**tenotomy** (tenotomía)
**testicle, testis** (testículo)
**testosterone** (testosterona)
**tetany** (tetania)
**thalamus** (tálamo)
**thalassemia** (talasemia)
**thoracocentesis** (toracocentesis)
**thoracostomy** (torascostomía)
**thorax** (tórax)
**throat** (garganta)
**throcotomy** (toracotomía)
**thrombectomy** (trombectomía)
**thrombin** (trombina)
**thrombocyte** (trombocito)
**thrombophlebitis** (tromboflebitis)
**thrombosis** (trombosis)
**thrombus** (trombo)
**thymectomy** (timectomía)
**thymoma** (timoma)
**thymosin** (timosina)
**thyroidectomy** (tiroidectomía)
**tibia** (tibia)
**tic** (tic)
**tinea** (tiña)
**tinnitus** (tinnitus)
**tongue** (lengua)
**tonometry** (tonometría)
**tonsillectomy** (tonsilectomía)
**tonsillitis** (tonsilitis)
**touch** (tacto)
**toxicology** (toxicología)
**trachea** (tráquea)
**tracheoplasty** (traqueoplastia)
**tracheostomy** (traquestomía)
**tracheotomy** (traqueotomía)
**traction** (tracción)
**transfusion** (transfusion)

tremor (temblor)
triglyceride (triglicérido)
trigone (trígono)
trochanter (trocánter)
trombolítico (thrombolytic)
tubercle (tubérculo)
tuberculosis (tuberculosis)
tuberosity (tuberosidad)
tumor (tumor)
tympanoplasty (timpanoplastia)

ulcer (úlcera)
ulna (ulna)
urea (urea)
uremia (uremia)
ureter (uréter)
urethra (uretra)
urinalysis (análisis de orina)
urine (orina)
urology (urología)
urticaria (urticaria)
uterus (útero)
uvea (úvea)
uvula (úvula)

vaccination (vacunación)
vaccine (vacuna)
vagina (vagina)
vaginitis (vaginitis)

valve (válvula)
valvulitis (valvulitis)
valvuloplasty (valvuloplastia)
varicella (varicela)
varicocele (varicocele)
vasectomy (vasectomía)
vasovasostomy (vasovasostomía)
vegetation (vegetación)
vein (vena)
venipuncture (venipuntura)
venography (venografía)
ventricle (ventrículo)
venule (vénula)
verruca, wart (verruga)
vertebra, pl. vertebrae (vertebra, pl. vertebras)
vertigo (vertigo)
vesicle (vesícula)
vestibule (vestíbule)
vial (vial)
villus (vellosidad)
virilism (virilismo)
vitamin (vitamina)
vitiligo (vitíligo)
volvulus (vólvulo)
vomer (vómer)
vulva (vulva)

wheal (roncha)
wheezes (sibilancia)

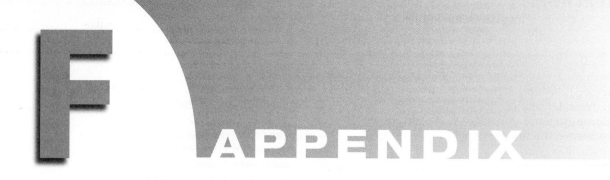

# Internet Resources

The selected list of Internet resources for allied health that follows is divided into allied health career organizations; government sites and resources; billing and insurance information; professional associations; and charitable organizations.

## Allied Health Careers

Anesthesiologist Assistant
American Academy of Anesthesiologists' Assistants (www.anesthestist.org)
Art Therapist
American Art Therapy Association (www.arttherapy.org)
Athletic Trainer
National Athletic Trainers' Association (www.nata.org)
Audiologist
American Speech-Language-Hearing Association (www.asha.org)
Blindness and Visual Impairment Professions
Association for Education and Rehilitation of the Blind and Visually Impaired (www.aerbvi.org)
Blood Bank Technology, Specialist in
American Society of Clinical Pathologists (www.ascp.org)
Cardiovascular Technologist
Society of Vascular Technologists (www.svtnet.org)
American Society of Echocardiography (www.asecho.org)
Alliance of Cardiovascular Professionals (www.acp-online.org)
Clinical Laboratory SciencëMedical Technology
American Society for Clinical Laboratory Science (www.alcls.org)
American Society for Clinical Pathology (www.ascp.org)
Association of Genetic Technologists (www.agt-info.org)
Counseling-related Occupations
American Counseling Association (www.counseling.org)
Cytotechnologist
American Society of Cytopathology (www.cytopathology.org)
Dental Assistant
American Dental Assistants Association (www.dentalassistant.org)
Dental Hygienist
American Dental Hygienists' Association (www.adha.org)
Dental Laboratory Technician
National Association of Dental Laboratories (www.nadl.org)
Diagnostic Medical Sonographer
Society of Diagnostic Medical Sonographers (www.sdms.org)
Dietetic Technician, Dietician
American Dietetic Association (www.eatright.org)

Electroneurodiagnostic Technology
American Society of Electroneurodiagnostic Technologists (www.aset.org)
Emergency Medical Technician-Paramedic
National Association of Emergency Medical Technicians (www.naemt.org)
Genetic Counselor
National Society of Genetic Counselors (www.nsgc.org)
Health Information Management
American Health Information Management Association  (www.ahima.org)
Histologic Technician/Histotechnologist
National Society for Histotechnology (www.nsh.org)
Kinesiotherapist
American Kinesiotherapy Association (www.akta.org)
Medical Assistant
American Association of Medical Assistants (www.aama-ntl.org)
Music Therapist
American Music Therapy Association (www.musictherapy.org)
Nuclear Medicine Technologist
Society of Nuclear Medicine — Technologist Section (http://interactivesnm.org)
Occupational Therapy
American Occupational Therapy Association (www.aota.org)
Ophthalmic Dispensing Optician
Opticians Association of America (www.opticians.org)
Opthalmic Laboratory Technician
Optical Laboratories Association (www.ola-labs.org)
Opthalmic Medical Technician/Technologist
Joint Commission on Allied Health Personnel in Opthalmology (www.jcahpo.org)
Orthoptist
American Orthoptic Council (www.orthoptics.org)
Orthotist and Prosthetic
American Orthotic and Prosthetic Association (www.aopanet.org)
Pathologists' Assistant
American Association of Pathologists' Assistants (www.pathologistsassistants.org)
Perfusionist
American Society of Extra-Corporeal Technologists (www.amsect.org)
Pharmacy Technician
American Association of Pharmacy Technicians (www.pharmacytechnician.com)
Physical Therapist, Physical Therapist Assistant
American Physical Therapy Association (www.apta.org)
Physician Assistant
American Academy of Physician Assistants (www.aapa.org)
Radiation Therapist, Radiographer
American Society of Radiologic Technologists (www.asrt.org)
Rehabilitation Counselor
National Rehabilitation Counseling Association (http://nrca-net.org)
Respiratory Therapist, Respiratory Therapy Technician
American Association for Respiratory Care (www.aarc.org)
Speech-Language Pathologist
American Speech-Language-Hearing Association (www.asha.org)
Surgical Assistant
National Surgical Assistant Association (www.nsaa.net)
Surgical Technologist
Association of Surgical Technologists (www.ast.org)

Therapeutic Recreation Specialist
American Therapeutic Recreation Association (www.atra-tr.org)

## Government Sites and Resources

**CDC**   Centers for Disease Control and Prevention (www.cdc.gov) links to many other sites set up by the CDC. For information, go to the main website and search for a specific subject or area and you will find the appropriate links.

**CCI**   The Medicare Correct Coding Initiative automated edits are online at
cms.hhs.gov/physicians/cciedits/default.asp

**CMS**   Coverage of the Centers for Medicare and Medicaid Services> Medicare, Medicaid, SCHIP, HIPAA, CLIA topics
www.cms.hhs.gov
Medicare Learning Network: cms.hhs.gov/mlngeninfo
Online Medicare manuals: cms.hhs.gov/manuals/IOM
Medicare Physician Fee Schedule: cms.hhs.gov/PhysicianFeeSchedule

**FDA**   Food and Drug Administration (www.fda.gov) is the main website for this agency with links to its many other websites.

**HCPCS**   General information on HCPCS
www.cms.hhs.gov/MedHCPCSGenInfo
Annual alphanumeric Healthcare Common Procedure Coding System file
www.cms.hhs.gov/HCPCSReleaseCodeSets

**SADMERC**
www.palmettogba.com

**HHS**   Health and Human Services (www.hhs.gov) is the main website for this agency with links to its many other websites.

**HIPAA**
Home page
www.cms.hhs.gov/hipaa/hipaa2/
Questions and Answers on HIPAA Privacy Policies
answers.hhs.gov

**HIPAA**   Privacy Rule
"Standards for Privacy of Individually Identifiable Health Information; Final Rule." 45 CFR Parts 160 and 164. *Federal Register 65*, no. 250 (2000).
www.hss.gov/ocr/hipaa/finalreg.html
ICD-9-CM addenda
www.cms.hhs.gov/ICD9ProviderDiagnosticCodes

**NCHS**   (National Center for Health Statistics) posts the ICD-9-CM addenda and guidelines
www.cdc.gov/nchs/datawh/ftpserv/ftpicd9/ftpicd9.htm guidelines

**NIH**   National Institutes for Health (www.nih.gov) is the main website for this agency with links to its many websites.

**NUBC**   The National Uniform Billing Committee develops and maintains a standardized data set for use by institutional providers to transmit claim and encounter information. This group is in charge of the 837I and the CMS-1450 (UB 04) claim formats.
www.nubc.org

**NUCC**   The National Uniform Claim Committee develops and maintains a standardized data set for use by the non-institutional health care community to transmit claim and encounter information. This group is in charge of the 837P and the CMS-1500 claim formats.
www.nucc.org

**OCR**   The Office of Civil Rights of the HHS enforces the HIPAA Privacy Rule; Privacy Fact Sheets are online at
www.hhs.gov/ocr/hipaa

**OIG**   The Office of Inspector General of the HHA home page links to fraud and abuse, advisory opinions, exclusion list, and other topics
www.oig.hhs.gov
Model compliance programs are found at
oig.hhs.gov/fraud/complianceguidance.html
TRICARE and CHAMPVA
General TRICARE information
www.tricare.osd.mil
CHAMPVA Overview
www.military.com/benefits/veterans-health-care/champva-overview
**WHO**   The International Statistical Classification of Diseases and Related Health Problems, tenth revision. is posted on the World Health Organization site
www.who.int/whosis/icd10/
**WPC**   Washington Publishing Company is the link for HIPAA Transaction and Code Sets implementation guides. It also assists several organizations in the maintenance and distribution of HIPAA-related code lists that are external to the X12 family of standards:

- Provider Taxonomy Codes
- Claim Adjustment Reason Codes
- Claim Status Codes
- Claim Status Category Codes
- Health Care Services Decision Reason Codes
- Insurance Business Process Application Error Codes
- Remittance Remark Codes

www.wpc-edi.com

## Billing and Insurance Resources

BlueCross BlueShield Association
www.bluecares.com
The Kaiser Family Foundation Web site provides in-depth information on key health policy issues such as Medicaid, Medicare, and prescription drugs.
www.kff.org
Various sites, such as www.benefitnews.com, www.erisaclaim.com and www.erisa.com, cover EMTALA, ERISA regulations and updates concerning provider and patient appeals of managed care organizations.
State insurance commissioners
www.omc.state.ct.us
**AHIMA**   Coverage of Related Topics Located Under the Practice Brief tab on the AHIMA Home Page
www.ahima.org
Computer-based Patient Record Institute (CPRI)
www.cpri.org
Medical Record Institute
www.medrecinst.com

## Professional Associations

**AADA**   American Dental Assistant Association (www.dentalassistants.org)
**AAFP**   American Academy of Family Physicians
www.aafp.org
**AAHAM**   American Association of Healthcare Administrative Management
www.aaham.org

**AAMA**  American Association of Medical Assistants
www.aama-ntl.org
**AAMT**  American Association for Medical Transcription (changing to Association for Integrity of Healthcare Documentation)
www.aamt.org
**AAPC**  American Academy of Professional Coders
www.aapc.com
**ACA**  American Chiropractic Association (**www.amerchiro.org**)
**ACA**  International (formerly American Collectors Association)
www.acainternational.org
**AHIP**  America's Health Plans
Links to Member Health Plans
www.ahip.org
**ACHE**  American College of Healthcare Executives
www.ache.org
**ADA**  American Dental Association (**www.ada.org**)
**ADHA**  American Dental Hygienists Association (**www.adha.org**)
**AHIMA**  American Health Information Management Association
www.ahima.org
**AMB**  Association of Medical Billers
www.billers.com
**AHLA**  American Health Lawyers Association
www.healthlawyers.org
**AHA**  American Hospital Association
www.aha.org
**AMA**  American Medical Association
www.ama-assn.org
**AMT**  American Medical Technologists
www.amt1.com
**AMTA**  American Massage Therapy Association (**www.amtamassage.org**)
**ANA**  American Nursing Association
www.ana.org
**APA**  American Psychiatric Association (**www.psych.org**)
**APTA**  American Physical Therapy Association (**www.apta.org**)
**CAMA**  Complementary Alternative Medicine Association (**www.camaweb.org**)
**HBMA**  Healthcare Billing and Management Association
www.hbma.com
**HFMA**  Healthcare Financial Management Association
www.hfma.org
**JCAHO**
**MGMA**  Medical Group Management Association
www.mgma.org
**PAHCOM**  Professional Association of Health Care Office Management
www.pahcom.com

## Charitable Organizations

AIDS.ORG (**www.aids.org**)
Alzheimer's Foundation of America (**www.alzfdn.org**)
American Cancer Society (**www.cancer.org**)
American Diabetes Association (**www.diabetes.org**)
American Heart Association (**www.americanheart.org**)

American Lung Association (www.lungusa.org)
Arthritis Foundation (www.arthritis.org)
Asthma and Allergy Foundation of America (www.aafa.org)
Cystic Fibrosis Foundation (www.cff.org)
The Leukemia and Lymphoma Society (www.leukemia-lymphoma.org)
National Multiple Sclerosis Society (www.nationalmssociety.org)
National Parkinson Foundation (www.parkinson.org)
Skin Cancer Foundation (www.skincancer.org)
United Cerebral Palsy (www.ucp.org)